Eat to Ease Osteoarthritis: 5 simple steps to reduce pain naturally

DISCLAIMER

All information in this book is intended to be used for general educational purposes only. This book is not intended to diagnose, treat, cure or prevent any medical conditions or diseases and should not be relied upon to replace medical advice or treatment. The information in this book is not medical advice and is not a substitute for medical treatment. You should consult a medical practitioner or other healthcare professional before making any changes to your diet or lifestyle.

The author accepts no responsibility for any loss or injury as a result of using/misusing any of the information contained in this book. Please consult a doctor or other qualified medical professional before taking any actions.

About the Author

Anne Pundak MSc is a musculo-skeletal specialist. She has been in private practice since 2000 and has helped thousands of patients suffering from pain including those suffering with arthritis. Anne Pundak received a Master's degree in Chiropractic in 2000 and has been running her own successful practice for the last 5 years in Buckinghamshire, England where she combines chiropractic treatment with nutritional and exercise advice.

Anne has a specific interest in nutrition since studying it as a topic while completing her degree. Through the years has become increasingly interested in the powerful health benefits of foods and their effects on our health. She has a passion for cooking, creating her own dishes and tasting local dishes from all around the world. She has travelled around the world, visiting local food markets and taking cooking courses to learn more about new ingredients and recipes.

Table of Contents

2

1. Introduction

If you are suffering from osteoarthritis, you have probably tried loads of different painkillers, medications and treatments to help ease your symptoms. It can be a minefield searching through the internet for information on how to relieve your symptoms. Especially when you are being presented with hundreds of different supplements, 'superfoods' or food plans which promise to 'cure' your arthritis. This vast amount of literature is overwhelming and makes it difficult to know what to try first.

At present, there is no for cure osteoarthritis. The search for a wonder drug to cure arthritis continues . . .

The good news is that there are a number of nutritional and lifestyle changes you can make to help reduce the pain caused by arthritis and help to prevent a rapid progression of symptoms.

The aim of this ebook is to:

Explain the cause and effects of osteoarthritis

Provide you with information you can use to improve your symptoms and quality of life through nutrition.

Having osteoarthritis (OA) can have a massive impact on your life due to the pain and restricted mobility associated with it. For some, the pain is debilitating and constant. It is tiring and depressing having to cope with trying to get through the day. This can be really hard to deal with especially if you have led a very active life and suddenly find yourself limited in what you can do

I believe that nutrition can play a huge part in relieving the symptoms of arthritis. Eating the right foods lowers the body's production of inflammation and reduces the build-up of nasty toxins around the joints.

Learning about how different foods affect your body will help you on your way to making better food choices so you can enjoy a greater state of well- being and health.

This book is designed to take you through a process of following simple steps to create and follow an eating plan which works for you. You will learn about what causes OA and how nutrition plays a fundamental role in reducing the inflammatory processes that cause and aggravate arthritic symptoms.

Food plays a vital role in preventing and managing many health conditions. Certain foods can aggravate arthritis whereas other foods fight against the inflammation and tissue destruction caused by arthritis.

Conventional medications used to treat OA often causes harmful side effects and their long-term use can actually increase inflammation in the body. There are many different dietary supplements aimed at arthritic pain but not all have been scientifically proven to be effective. Research and studies on supplements and herbs is readily available. In some cases their effectiveness can prove inconclusive or ineffective. However, there are studies which have shown that many OA sufferers have found significant relief when using certain herbs and supplements. It is important to know what good quality scientific research has demonstrated regarding their safety and effectiveness.

Managing OA is complicated as every individual has their symptoms and respond differently to various foods and supplements. Claims of a perfect diet, supplement or superfood which suits every single arthritis sufferer is not realistic and won't cure your arthritis. What works for one person doesn't work for another person because we are all different.

As individuals, our genetic and biochemical make-up is unique to ourselves. This means that we all have different nutritional needs in terms of how much we need to eat and what we need to eat. Our lifestyles and our exposure to different environmental toxins also varies. All these factors can affect the development of conditions such as arthritis as you will learn later.

There is no miracle diet that will cure OA. You need to be wary of diets claiming to cure or eliminate all symptoms. Everyone responds differently to different foods and supplements so there is no 'one diet fits all' plan. This guide introduces you to the basic principles of including anti-inflammatory foods which have been found to be beneficial in reducing symptoms of osteoarthritis.

2. How can you benefit from the healing effects of food?

The body possesses its own 'innate' power to heal itself which means that the power to heal is within you. What you eat and put in your body plays a crucial role in how healthy you are and how you can support your body's own innate mechanism to heal itself.

Changing your diet will allow you to start making steady progress towards and healing and restoring your body.

The Link between Food and Health

Studies have shown that there is a relationship between food and health that goes beyond it being just a source of energy. We know that foods are made up of carbohydrates, protein and fats and some foods provide us with essential vitamins and minerals. But that's not where it stops.

There are nutrients in food that act on the body's chemical pathways on a molecular level. These pathways are responsible for all aspects of our body's functioning. There are certain foods which contain nutrients that are able to trigger diseases while others have a healing effect that actually prevent diseases from occurring.

Natural anti-inflammatory compounds found in food have been found to reduce the swelling and pain associated with OA, while other nutrients are able to supply the underlying building blocks of joints and reduce damage caused to the joint cartilage

Therefore eating natural unprocessed food rich in disease-preventing nutrients is crucial in triggering our own internal healing mechanisms to get better and prevent diseases from occurring.

3. What is Osteoarthritis?

It is a degenerative arthritis and the most common form of arthritis. It is caused by the breakdown and loss of the cartilage between a joint. In particular, it affects the hands, neck, low back, knees and hips

Normal Joint Anatomy

We will be referring to synovial or articular joints which are the joints affected by osteoarthritis. A **joint** is where 2 bones connect to each other. Its function is to allow movement and provide support.

In a healthy joint, the ends of bones are covered by smooth cartilage which reduces the friction between the bones as they move. The whole joint is covered with a tissue called the synovial membrane, which secretes synovial fluid.

Synovial fluid lubricates the cartilage and makes sure that the joint continues to move smoothly.

It has two main functions:

- It lubricates the joint and cartilage - allowing the joints to glide smoothly over one another.

- It supplies nutrients to the cartilage and removes waste products that build up in the joint.

So we know that osteoarthritis is caused by the breakdown of the joint cartilage but what is cartilage and what does it do?

What is joint cartilage?

The cartilage that lines our joints is called **articular cartilage**. It is a tough but flexible type of connective tissue which lines the ends of the bones that form our joints.

It is primarily made up of 3 components:

- **Water**: 70-80%

- **Collagen Fibres:** 10-15%

- **Proteoglycans:** 5-10%

Water

Joint cartilage is mainly made up of water. Joints are able to withstand extremely high levels of pressure by releasing water from the cartilage.

Collagen and Proteoglycans

They provide the strength and support to the cartilage and are designed to absorb any pressure or load which is exerted through the joint.

Why is Cartilage Important?

- It provides cushioning within the joints and acts like a shock absorber.

-It prevents our bones from grinding and rubbing against each other during movement.

In a Nutshell

Cartilage is a smooth surface which reduces friction to a bare minimum during movement. Movement of the joints increases the production of synovial fluid. In turn the synovial fluid keeps cartilage healthy by reducing friction.

How Does Cartilage Stay Healthy?

Unfortunately cartilage does not have a direct blood supply unlike most other tissues in the body. The blood vessels stop at the edge of the cartilage and do not carry nutrients deep into the cartilage. Our cartilage receives its nutrients through a process called imbibition.

Motion is Lotion

Movement is the key to good joint nutrition. Imbibition refers to the exchange of fluid via movement. The compressive and flexion/extension forces exerted on the joint through movement create a pumping action which keeps fluids flowing into the cartilage. This serves to pump in nutrients like oxygen and glucose (sugars). This pumping action also removes waste products such as carbon dioxide.

Osteoarthritis Damages Cartilage and Bone

Cartilage is a very difficult tissue to repair and rebuild. Chondrocytes, (the cells that make collagen and proteoglycans) can stop working properly. The cartilage holds on to water and begins to swell. As the cartilage swells up it becomes soft and begins to break down. The bone underneath the cartilage can start to erode. This erosion leads to an uneven, rough surface. The cartilage becomes thinner as the repair of cartilage cannot keep up with its destruction. As it becomes thinner, the cartilage cannot absorb shock as well and becomes more susceptible to damage

Damaged cartilage is often associated with damage to the bone beneath the cartilage:
As the cartilage breaks down and begins to wear away, the bones underneath begin to rub against each other. In the final stages, the cartilage becomes rough and uneven. Bits of cartilage and bone can begin to breakdown and float inside the joint leading to more pain and swelling. Over time, the joint may also become misshapen.

Osteophytes – Bone Spurs

Bone spurs called osteophytes can begin to grow around the edges of the joint. A bone spur forms as the body tries to repair itself by building extra bone. Osteophytes usually form when bone is subjected to prolonged pressure, rubbing, or stress.

These bony changes can be the result of altered spinal biomechanics such as lack of movement or joint misalignment. Osteophytes can cause wear and tear or pain if they press or rub on other bones or soft tissues (such as ligaments, tendons, or nerves).

Symptoms of Osteoarthritis

The rubbing of bones against each other as they move causes pain, swelling, stiffness and loss of joint movement. - Typically, the pain is aggravated by using the joint and relieved by rest. However, as the disease worsens, the pain becomes more constant.

Symptoms include:

- Swelling , pain, stiffness and warmth in one or more joints

- A grinding, clicking or cracking sensation when the joint is moved

- Stiffness in a joint after sitting or lying for a long time

- Loss of muscle mass and weakness around affected joint

Diagnosis

OA is diagnosed by taking a medical history, performing a physical examination and taking x-rays or MRI scans.

4. Causes of Osteoarthritis

The exact cause of OA is not clearly understood. There are a number of risk factors that are known to increase the likelihood of developing OA.

Age

Age is the main and primary risk factor in developing OA. Usually OA sufferers are over the age of 40. It can affect younger individuals but is rare. As we get older, articular cartilage begins to degenerate. The number of proteoglycans in our cartilage reduces as we get older. This leads to the deterioration of the cartilage.

Obesity

Excess weight adds extra pressure onto weight-bearing joints. Your hips and knees are major weight-bearing joints. Being overweight puts extra pressure on these joints. Years of carrying an extra load can cause the cartilage to break down. Obesity can cause osteoarthritis to develop on its own, or in combination with other factors can worsen the severity of arthritis.

Trauma

Joint cartilage is a complicated tissue that has a limited capacity of repair. Trauma is a major cause of destruction of cartilage. It is a high risk factor in developing OA in the affected joint Sustained repetitive movements or serious injuries to joints (surgery, fractures) can lead to the onset of osteoarthritis.

Sports can damage or cause repetitive stress to joints, tendons and ligaments, can speed up the breakdown of cartilage. Even low weight-bearing joints like the shoulder can become arthritic if it is subjected to injuries or repetitive stress.

Activity Levels

There is a fine balance in keeping fit and active. Too much or too little activity can affect your joints. A lack of movement and exercise leads to weaker muscles and joints that can become stiff and painful. Too much exercise especially the high-impact type can cause repetitive stress and trauma to your joints.

Genetics

In certain families, several members develop osteoarthritis leading to suggestion that there is a genetic predisposition in developing arthritis. However, genes responsible for triggering arthritis have not been identified. One theory is that some people may have a defect in the gene responsible for the collagen production. This uncommon genetic defect could lead to weaker cartilage that wears down after a few decades of regular activity, and could explain why osteoarthritis is sometimes seen in people as young as twenty.

Gout

With gout, the body produces an excessive amount of uric acid crystals which can become deposited inside joints and cause damage to the cartilage

Smoking

It is thought that smoking can trigger cartilage loss. Also, **smoking seems to trigger OA in younger people.** OA sufferers who smoke are more likely to suffer from more pain than non-smokers who have OA. Osteoarthritis sufferers who smoke larger number of cigarettes can more severe joint problems. While OA tends to affect people as they get older

Allergies/Food Intolerance:

They can lead to persistent chronic inflammation which can weaken the immune system. Continuous raised levels of inflammation can eventually damage joints.

In a Nutshell

The cause of OA is still not fully understood but certain factors increasing the chances of developing OA have been identified. Some of these factors such as your age, genetics or previous trauma are beyond your control. Other factors are linked to your lifestyle and are controllable. These factors include your weight, activity levels and diet and you have the ability to modify them.

5. Conventional Medication

Conventional medications have been shown to provide pain relief from the symptoms caused by OA. But when used regularly and over long periods of time (chronic use), they are associated with a range of side effects of which some are very serious. These include headaches, dizziness, cartilage destruction, cardiovascular symptoms, gastrointestinal irritation/damage and kidney or liver damage.

NSAID's – Non-Steroidal Anti-Inflammatories

These drugs are the main medications used to manage arthritis. Over-the-counter NSAIDs (such as ibuprofen and naproxen) work by blocking the cyclooxygenase enzymes (COX-1 and COX-2. COX-1 and COX-2 enzymes are major causes of joint inflammation and pain. They work by converting arachidonic acid into prostaglandins.

Prostaglandins are hormone like substances that promote inflammation and influence pain signals - causing pain, redness and swelling during the inflammatory process.

Risks:

Can cause upsets of the gastrointestinal tract and long term use can cause gastrointestinal bleeding. Regular use of NSAIDs, gives you 3 times the risk of developing serious gastrointestinal side effects than those who don't use them.

Certain NSAIDs have been removed from circulation due to the increased risk of cardiovascular events such as heart attacks. Also, many people with chronic pain find their medication irritates their stomach causing ulcers and bleeding. More people die each year as a result of peptic ulcers caused by anti-inflammatory medications than from cocaine abuse [1].

Using NSAIDs can speed up the destruction of the joint cartilage [2]. Studies have shown that the use of NSAID's over a long period of time significantly increases the risk of cartilage breakdown [3].

Corticosteroids

They are primarily used as a treatment for rheumatoid arthritis. In severe cases of osteoarthritis, steroids are injected directly into the painful joint. Corticosteroids have significant risks associated with their use. Caution must be used when taking them.
Injections are generally spaced months apart to avoid joint damage and degeneration.

Risks:

Long-term oral corticosteroid use is associated with a wide range of effects, including weight gain, osteoporosis, stress fractures and adrenal gland failure [4].

Painkillers (Analgesics)

Paracetamol

Paracetamol is an analgesic which means it works as a painkiller. It is not classed as an NSAID as it has very weak anti-inflammatory properties. This drug is easily available over the counter.

Risks:

Long term use of paracetamol can cause upper gastro-intestinal (stomach) bleeding and liver toxicity [5].

Opiod Analgesics

Opiod analgesics such as codeine, tramadol and morphine are sometimes used to control pain in severe and acute flare-ups of osteoarthritis.

Risks:

They must only be used for short periods because of the risk of dependency.

Side effects of morphine and codeine include constipation, nausea, vomiting, dizziness and drowsiness. Side effects associated with tramadol include a feeling of fuzzy-headedness and confusion [6,7].

In a Nutshell

Medications are the conventional treatment used for reducing the symptoms of OA. However they are associated with many side effects, many of which can be serious particularly with long-term use of these medications. More worryingly, some of the medications used to relieve the OA symptoms actually worsen the progression of this disease by damaging the cartilage and joints.

6. Nutrition on a Molecular Level

The goal of eating well is to provide the body with the specific nutrients it requires to function at an optimal level. Studies have shown that foods interact with particular genes and can increase the likelihood of developing chronic diseases. Nutrients act on a molecular level and can affect health by changing gene structure and expression. The effects of what you eat on your health depend on your genetic make-up. None of us are genetically identical —we are all unique.

Taking care of Our Cells

Our cells are the building blocks of our body. They are working at their most efficient levels when we are in good health. Cells breakdown and remove waste products that accumulate in our bodies. Cells are constantly dividing into 2 new but identical cells – this process is called cell replication which is essential when it comes to repairing the body's tissues.

Genes and DNA

Our cells contain our DNA. DNA can be described as your own personal database that contains all the information about you in the form of a code. Our genes store this information or code (called genetic information) in the form of strands called DNA. We all have our own unique information which our genes express.

For example: a gene contains a code for a specific protein. A protein's job is to perform a particular function: ie: the amylase protein performs a chemical reaction to break down starches in the foods that we eat. Genes can be switched on or off – a process called gene expression.

When a gene is switched on, a portion of the code in that gene is read to make a protein. Once that protein is made, the gene is 'switched' off. Switching on a gene triggers a process which allows a particular protein to be made.

DNA Damage

DNA can also be damaged and once damaged only has a limited capacity to repair. When cells replicate, the new cells also carry the same DNA damage which in the long term can result in the development of diseases.

It's in the genes

We are born with genes that contain DNA that have the potential to make us more likely to develop certain illnesses. However, research has shown us that the way our genes express this information can be controlled. You can carry genes that code for arthritis or heart disease. But just because you carry that gene – does not necessarily mean that you will get that disease. This is because the gene needs to be switched on before the condition can develop.

Pushing the Switch

Environment triggers and lifestyle choices have the power to switch genes on or off. Stress levels, exposure to toxins (environmental pollutants, cleaning chemicals, trauma and what we eat can affect whether or not these genes are activated. They are able to alter the structure of our DNA and control what gets expressed through a process called methylation.

Food and Genes

Foods can interact with our genes and have an influence on how they are expressed. Studies have shown that food is a powerful factor in determining whether disease-causing genes are on or off. Nutrients are so powerful that eating the right foods can actually undo the damage that chemical and environmental toxins cause to our genes. Now that's food for thought [8].

In a Nutshell

You have learned that our genes can predispose us to develop illnesses. Nutrition and environmental factors are major players in determining if we ever develop these diseases. Poor diet choices can result in us suffering from health problems. However, food is so powerful in controlling gene expression, that making the right choices can actually influence whether or not those genes are switched on.

7. The Relevance of Chronic Inflammation in the Management of Osteoarthritis

What is Inflammation?

Inflammation is the body's response to injury. It describes the process in which white blood cells and chemicals are released to protect and repair the body from infection or injury. An acute inflammatory (controlled and short) response is essential in order for the body to heal itself from damage. Once the damage is repaired, the process of inflammation shuts off.

Chronic Inflammation

However, inflammation can become chronic when having to fight off long-term or repeated stress and cannot turn itself off. Over time the body will becomes overstressed as it weakens from having to continually fight. This weakens the immune system which makes the body more susceptible to developing chronic diseases. Chronic inflammation is not easily detected – it can be symptomless or present with vague symptoms such as lack of energy.

Interestingly, inflammation is connected to obesity – and obesity to arthritis – because fat cells can produce cytokines – cytokines are proteins that encourage inflammation.

Causes of Chronic Inflammation

Inflammation becomes chronic (long-lasting) when there is persistent long-term stimulation

Chronic inflammation can be caused by one or more of the following:

- **Foods** – processed, refined foods

- **Toxins** – heavy metals, chemicals, pesticides, smoking, food additives

- **Allergens/food intolerances**

- **Persistent old injuries or infections** - cause low levels of inflammation to persist

- **Stress -** the hormones produced during a stress response use and deplete essential minerals. Prolonged periods of stress cause acidic conditions which promote inflammatory processes.

Diseases occur as a result of the release of inflammatory chemicals that affect body tissues. There is a lot of research which is beginning to show a link between inflammation and the development of many chronic diseases such as: **cancer, type 2 diabetes, arthritis, heart disease, inflammatory bowel disease, hormonal imbalances, allergies and asthma to name but a few** [9].

Free Radicals

Free radicals are produced in the body during normal metabolic processes such as breaking down food. They are also produced by the immune system in response to an injury or infection and promote healing.

Free radicals are unstable molecules which cause tissue damage through a process called oxidative stress. Free radicals attack other molecules that then become unstable too. These molecules go on to attack other molecules and keep the cycle going.

Chronic inflammation leads to an overproduction of free radicals by the immune system which can lead to developing inflammatory related diseases. Increased levels of free radicals build up in the body when you are exposed to pollution, cigarette smoke, radiation and chemicals or eat certain foods.

Research has shown that oxidative stress plays a role in the development of OA. During oxidative stress, high levels of free radicals build up and cause damage to the body's tissues [10].

Fighting Free Radicals

In OA, free radicals can circulate within the fluid of the joints. This damages the joint lining, allowing the fluid to leak out. This in turn reduces the shock absorbency capability of the affected joint.

The accumulation of free radicals in joints also causes swelling and degeneration of the joint and cartilage.

The good news is that your body is equipped to handle free radicals. Antioxidants protect the body from the damage caused by free radicals by neutralizing them. Vitamins A, C and E (ACE) are powerful anti-oxidants. Antioxidants are vitamins and other substances that supply missing electrons for unstable molecules in order to prevent free radical damage

In a Nutshell

Inflammation is a natural response to injury or infections. However when it becomes chronic due to other underlying factors, it can become harmful because it can cause pain and illnesses. The effects of chronic inflammation, free radical damage and oxidative stress have become major topics of research due to their harmful impact on the body. Chronic inflammation can lead to the onset of a many types of diseases and conditions such as cancer, cardiovascular disease, type 2 diabetes, hormonal imbalances, inflammatory bowel disease (IBD), rheumatoid arthritis and osteoarthritis.

8. Natural Management of Osteoarthritis

Cartilage is difficult to repair, which is why it is so important to reduce the levels of inflammatory molecules in the body. This is why it is crucial to pay attention to diet, nutrition, exercise, stress management and body weight.

Natural anti-inflammatories found in our food are safer and more effective than medications. Nutrients have a greater capacity to tone down a wider range of inflammatory processes whereas a drug can only affect one specific molecule in one process.

The Good News…….

Your body is fully capable of rebuilding cartilage and synovial fluid, but in order to effectively do so it needs the proper building blocks.

Nutritional Goals: 5 Simple Steps to Reduce Pain Naturally

1. Reduce foods that promote inflammation in the body

2. Introduce foods that are anti-inflammatory into your diet

3. Keep your blood sugar levels balanced

4. Eliminate anti-arthritic foods

5. Add herbs and supplements that reduce joint inflammation and support cartilage

You now know that chronic inflammation is a damaging process. Therefore the first step in managing your arthritic symptoms is to gain knowledge of both harmful and beneficial foods and nutrients.

Firstly you need to know which foods:

Cause inflammation and aggravate osteoarthritis

Heal and possess anti-inflammatory actions that can ease the symptoms of OA

9. STEP 1 - Reduce foods that promote inflammation in the body

Inflammatory Foods

There are certain foods, preservatives and additives that increase inflammation in the body. The following information will guide you on which foods to eliminate or reduce.

Refined Carbohydrates

Refined carbs are unhealthy. They have been processed to strip away their fibre content. They are found in white flour and sugars. These foods contain calories but are low in nutrients. They are high on the glycemic index – which means that they rapidly spike up your blood sugar levels and increases levels of inflammation. More information about the glycemic index of foods will be covered later on.

Foods to Avoid:

White breads, pastas and white rice.

Refined white sugars, corn syrup, cane sugar

Refined sugars are found in soft drinks, sweetened coffee and tea drinks, milkshakes and certain breakfast cereals, biscuits, cakes, sweets and pastries. A lot of fat free or reduced fat foods such as yogurts and ready meals contain higher levels of sugars and sweeteners - despite being labelled as healthier due to reduced fat levels [11].

Trans Fats

Trans Fats are hydrogenated vegetable oils. They block the use of essential fatty acids - while increasing the level of bad cholesterol. They also cause inflammation by causing immune system dysfunction.

Foods to Avoid:

Margarines, shortenings, pastries, fast foods, processed foods and crisps (potato chips) as they all contain high levels.

*A lot of food companies are now reducing or eliminating trans fats from their products so look out for this on food labels.

**Alternatives to trans fats include small amounts of butter/lard, coconut oil, palm oil and mono-unsaturated vegetable oils such as olive and avocado oil.

Unhealthy Fats

- Avoid margarine and spreads

- Avoid skimmed cheeses, low fat yogurts and soya based products

- Avoid hydrogenated or partially hydrogenated fats

- Avoid corn, soy, safflower, sunflower and rapeseed (canola) oils as they can contain toxic chemicals and are high in omega 6's

- Avoid ready- made salad dressings as they can be high in sugar and processed vegetable oils.

Foods High in Arachidonic Acid

Arachidonic acid is an essential fatty acid in the omega 6 family. It is necessary for muscle tissue growth. However, in higher levels, it has been found to increase inflammation and pain in joints.

Another note on meat:

*Supermarket milks and meats contain steroids, antibiotics and hormones which are unnatural and disrupt the proper functioning of our immune system – in turn promoting inflammation. Find out where you can buy grass fed, free-range organic meats/milk – it is worth eating less meat but paying more for a cut of meat which is healthier [12].

Foods to reduce:

- Meat – especially red meat

- Milk – cows are fed high levels of grain which contain high levels of Omega 6 fats

- Cheese

- Eggs

Higher levels of arachidonic acid are found in red meats, offal (organ meats) and egg yolks

Arthritis sufferers are recommended to reduce meat and eat more fish.

Coffee/Tea/Soft Drinks

Coffee and black tea are acidic. Acidity is a major cause of inflammation. Be aware that apart from being high in sugar, soft drinks also contain phosphoric acid. Phosphoric acid weakens bones by depleting bones and teeth from minerals including calcium [13].

Alcohol

Alcohol promotes inflammation. It also flushes out vital nutrients and B vitamins. Long-term excessive use of alcohol can cause bones to thin causing bone loss and destruction. Due to the dehydrating effects of alcohol, muscles can become stiffer leading to even more discomfort [14].

Vegetables from the nightshade family

They contain steroid alkaloids that can lead to increased inflammation, muscle spasm, pain and stiffness. Alkaloids also interfere with new formation of cartilage and block it from repairing. **Nighshades includes: Tomatoes, Red, Green and Yellow Peppers (not black pepper), Hot Chillies, White Potatoes, Tobacco, Aubergines (eggplants)**

It is important to mention that edible vegetables in the nightshade family contain low levels experts state there are no studies confirming that the exclusion of nightshade vegetables from the diet improves arthritic symptoms.

However, there are couple of studies which have reported pain relief when osteoarthritis sufferers eliminated/reduced these vegetables from their diet. Those that reported relief often obtained significant levels of pain relief.

A study in 1993 showed that out of 5000 people who avoided nightshade vegetables, 70% reported a significant reduction in pain [15]. Another study showed improvement in symptoms in 1400 patients who were observed over a 20 year period [16].

*Note: green tomatoes, green peppers and green parts on potatoes contain higher levels of alkaloids. Make sure to cut out any green parts of flesh or skin of a potato.

Preservatives, Additives and Sweeteners

Avoid ready- made meals and foods containing sweeteners, additives and preservatives. They are often found in foods that have a low nutritional value. They are made up of chemical compounds that can create sensitivities in certain individuals and have the capability to worsen underlying health conditions. They can be toxic and inflammatory and are linked to the development of certain illnesses including cancers [17].

Processed Foods

Eliminate processed foods as they are cooked at a high temperature to give them a long shelf life and contain AGES, synthetic chemicals and preservatives

Processed foods contain a lot of unhealthy chemicals. They tend to be high in trans fats, salt, sugar, high-fructose corn syrup and synthetic flavourings. Avoid or even better eliminate the following foods:

- Processed meats: bacon, sausages, lunch meats (ham, salami, pates)
- Cookies, cakes, pastries
- Crisps
- Ready meals
- Low-fat and fat-free foods
- Fast food/take-aways

In a Nutshell

There are certain foods which are classed as being pro-inflammatory agents. These include highly processed foods, refined carbohydrates and foods that are high in sugar, omega 6's or arachidonic acids. These foods are able to create inflammation through their involvement in complex biomechanical processes in the body that create inflammation.

10. Step 2 - Introduce foods that are anti-inflammatory into your diet

So what foods can you eat?

It wasn't so long ago that people regularly ate butter, eggs and meats – diets which were high in fats and cholesterol. However there was a lower incidence of health conditions caused by chronic inflammation. A major factor was that they were not exposed to fast food, processed foods, additives and preservatives. The food they ate was local, unprocessed and additive-free.

You want to introduce foods that are anti-inflammatory. Vegetables, fruits, herbs, spices are loaded with powerful anti-inflammatory and antioxidant properties. Foods rich in omega 3's reduce inflammation. Eating foods with a lower glycaemic load keep your blood sugar levels balanced and reduce inflammatory effects.

Omega 3 Fatty Acids

They are the building blocks of many anti-inflammatory compounds in the body. Most western diets are **low in omega 3** and contain a **higher ratio of Omega 6 to Omega 3.** Omega 3's reduces inflammation and joint stiffness. Many clinical studies have proved the value of omega-3 fatty acids in treating inflammatory conditions.

Omega-3 fatty acids have been shown in some studies to reduce the pain of osteoarthritis. When the diet contains plenty of these essential fats, the cells make less pro-inflammatory substances and more anti-inflammatory substances. These fats work by reducing inflammation which prevent the damage to the cartilage and connective tissue that usually occurs in osteoarthritis [18].

Foods rich in Omega 3 Fatty Acids

- Fish such as trout, wild salmon, mackerel, sardines and herring

- Flaxseed, sesame seeds, pumpkin seeds, pecans, brazil nuts, almonds, walnuts

The most potent of the omega-3 fatty acids are:

- Eicosapentaenoic Acid (EPA)

- Docosahexaenoic Acid (DHA)

The effectiveness of EPA and DHA fatty acids are increased if foods rich in omega-6 are kept to a minimum.

Fat Breakdown

Our body breaks fats down to their basic components through a series of chemical processes. When broken down, certain fats produce prostaglandins (PG's). Some prostaglandins are anti-inflammatory and reduce pain and inflammation while other types of prostaglandins actually promote inflammatory responses. It is important to maintain a balance between the anti-inflammatory and pro-inflammatory PG's

Omega 6 Fatty Acids

Omega 3 fats are a great source for producing good anti-inflammatory PG's whereas Omega 6 fats promote pro-inflammatory PG production [19]. Omega-6 fatty acids are found in: corn, sunflower and safflower oils (which are regularly found in snack foods), fried foods, margarines, spreads, meat and eggs.

Omega 3 versus Omega 6

Studies have shown that Cox-2 enzymes become more active leading to more joint inflammation when a diet is higher in omega-6 fatty acids than omega-3 fatty acids. The majority of people consume approximately 10 times Omega-6's than Omega-3's [20].

Having a high Omega 6 to Omega 3 ratio disrupts prostaglandin levels. Balancing our prostaglandin levels helps to stop chronic inflammation staying in our bodies. Omega-6 fatty acids increase inflammation which can add to the pain and stiffness of osteoarthritis. Eating increased amounts of omega-3 fatty acids and decreasing your intake of omega-6 fatty acids) can improve symptoms and may allow you to reduce pain medications [21].

A nutritional daily recommended dose for Omega 3 has not been established but experts have suggested consuming 3 grams per day. 2 tbsp of flaxseed oil contain 3.5g while a 3.5 oz piece of fish contains 1g. For general health, two 3-ounce servings of fish a week are recommended. However, it's difficult to get the recommended dose of Omega-3's from simply eating fish.

Adding a fish oil supplement to your diet can be a good way of getting a good dose of Omega-3's into your diet [22, 23].

Fish Oils

They contain a concentrated source of the omega 3 fatty acid called **eicosapaentanoic acid (EPA)** which can significantly reduce inflammation. Only use high quality, purified fish oils. To treat arthritis-related conditions, use fish oil capsules containing 1,400 mg of EPA and 1000 mg of DHA daily [24].

Anti-Oxidants

Anti-oxidants reduce the damage from the inflammatory effect caused by free radicals. They work by neutralising these radicals. Our bodies can make anti-oxidants - **ACE vitamins** are loaded with antioxidants. As we age, the production of antioxidant enzymes gradually decreases. Vitamins are essential nutrients found in vegetables and fruits.

The ACE/Selenium Combination

Vitamin A

It is a powerful free radical scavenger which helps promote normal bone development. It is a powerful antioxidant that helps reduce the risk of the effects of osteoarthritis. Studies have shown that a diet rich in beta-carotenes slows down the progression of osteoarthritis [25]. **Beta carotene** is found in red, yellow and orange fruits and vegetables and is converted into vitamin A in the body.

Think colours when selecting veggies and fruit rich in beta-carotene: carrots, squashes, sweet potatoes, pumpkin, peppers, apricots and cantaloupes. Lots of dark-green leafy vegetables such as spinach, kale and romaine lettuce also contain beta-carotene.

Vitamin C

This vitamin is a very powerful antioxidant in the body. It works by neutralizing free radicals, which helps reduce the inflammation and damage that occurs in osteoarthritis.

Vitamin C is also necessary for the production of healthy connective tissue and cartilage.
It also plays an essential role in the repair and maintenance of cartilage. Vitamin C is required to form collagen (collagen is an important protein used to make tendons, cartilage, ligaments, skin and blood vessels).

Vitamin C may even be able to help undo some of the cartilage damage that has already been done by the arthritic process. The progression of OA appears to be slower in individuals who have diets rich in vitamin C in their diet [26].

Excellent food sources of vitamin C include: broccoli, parsley, bell peppers, strawberries, cauliflower, lemons, mustard greens, Brussels sprouts, papaya, kale, cabbage, spinach, kiwifruit, cantaloupe, oranges, grapefruit, tomatoes, chard, collard greens, raspberries, peppermint leaves, asparagus, celery, fennel bulb, pineapple, and watermelon.

Note: extremely high levels of vitamin C can speed up cartilage damage in osteoarthritis sufferers.
The recommended dose for adults is between 75 mg (women) and 90 mg (men) of vitamin C each day [27].

40

Vitamin E

The anti-oxidants in vitamin E have a significant effect in protecting cartilage from damage by eliminating cartilage-damaging free radicals. It is also very good at reducing inflammation - which provides pain relief and improves joint mobility.

Studies have shown that osteoarthritis sufferers with a good intake of vitamin E report a significant reduction in their pain. Many are even able to reduce the amount of pain-killers they need to take [28].

Almonds, sunflower seeds, chard and mustard greens are a few excellent sources of vitamin E.

Selenium

This mineral is a component of an anti-oxidant enzyme which blocks free radicals. Good sources of selenium are found in brazil nuts, fish/seafood, poultry, meats, brown rice, oats and wholegrains. Selenium works better when combined with Vitamin E as it enhances its effectiveness [29].

Anti-Oxidant Rich Foods

Vegetables, fruits, nuts seeds, pulses and legumes contain high levels of anti-oxidants. It is more beneficial to get your source of anti-oxidants naturally through foods rather than supplements. Synthetic antioxidants are not as beneficial as naturally occurring anti-oxidants.

Leafy greens and green vegetables

Greens are bursting full of antioxidants which neutralize the effects of free radicals which create joint damage created by persistent chronic inflammation.

Leafy greens include lettuces, rocket, kale, spinach, watercress, pak choi, cabbages, endives

Green veggies include asparagus, brussel sprouts, broccoli, artichokes, green beans, celery, chards and peas.

Green Smoothies

Green smoothies are a delicious way to get more out of the nutrients found in leafy greens and fruits. Leafy greens contain high levels of ACE vitamins as well as numerous anti-inflammatory combines.

Green smoothies are made by blending fresh greens with fresh fruit in a smoothie maker or blender. It is recommended to have a higher ratio of greens to fruit (about 60% greens to 40% fruit).

Leafy greens are hard to digest as it is difficult to chew them down to a creamy consistency.

Blending the greens breaks them down and they are consumed in a more pre-digested state - therefore releasing more nutrients than if you were to eat them whole.

Benefits include:

- Weight loss as cravings for sugar and junk food are reduced
- They fill you up

- Increase your amount of green vegetables and fruit intake

- Increase levels of antioxidants

- Increase your Energy levels

- Increase your fibre intake

- Anti-inflammatory

*Note - Drinking green smoothies shouldn't be a replacement for eating whole greens and whole greens should still be incorporated into your diet.

Blend:

- Leafy greens: spinach, kale and romaine lettuce.
- Fruits: apples, avocados, blueberries, cherries, strawberries, mango, pineapple, pears and bananas.

You can experiment using different combinations of greens and fruits, using whatever combinations you feel like. Add enough water in the blender so that when the greens and fruits are combined, they blend down to a smoothie-like consistency.

For an extra anti-oxidant and anti-inflammatory effect: add spices like cinnamon or chilli, flaxseed oil or a squirt of lemon juice.

Wholegrains

Your body digests wholegrains slowly, which keep your blood sugar levels stable.

Whole grains lower levels by up to 40% of C-reactive protein (CRP) in the blood, a marker of inflammation [30].

They also contain fibre which helps to fill you up and promote weight loss. Wheat and oats almost equal broccoli and spinach in antioxidant activity [31].

Foods Sources:

Brown rice is recommended. Other wholegrains to try are oats, rye, barley, millett and wholewheat. To increase grains in your diet, try eating oatmeal, brown rice, whole-grain cereal and whole-wheat crackers – all foods where the majority of the grain comes from whole grain.

Pasta – wholewheat pasta or rice/buckwheat noodles are recommended. Cooking pasta 'al dente' reduces the GI load.

Legumes and Pulses

They are rich in protein and fibre, have a low glycemic index and rich in anti-oxidants making them an ideal food to include in your food plan.

Good sources include kidney beans, chick peas, cannellini beans, pinto beans and lentils. Add them to salads, soups, curries and stews or blend them into spreads or dips.

When using tinned varieties make sure they have a low salt and sugar content and always rinse them before eating.

Anti-Arthritic Super Foods

Plant-based foods contain antioxidants and phytochemicals, which can decrease many pro-inflammatory substances in the body that help to reduce joint inflammation and support cartilage repair.

1. Berries

Berries are packed with antioxidants such as vitamin C. Brightly coloured berries contain more beta-carotene. Berries also contain an anti-inflammatory agent called **quercetin** [32]. Strawberries, raspberries, blueberries and cranberries are great berries to add to your diet.

2. Broccoli

A compound in broccoli called **sulforaphane,** could prevent cartilage from breaking down, by blocking the action of cartilage-degrading enzymes, according to a study done by Ian Clark, PhD, a professor in the University of East Anglia's School of Biological Sciences.

He hopes to learn whether, when broccoli is eaten regularly, does "sulforaphane actually gets into the joint and cartilage at appropriate doses to display activity [in the body]," he says [33]. Sulforaphane is also found in brussel sprouts, cabbage, kale and cauliflowers.

3. Cherries

Cherries are rich in antioxidants, including **quercetin,** vitamin C, and beta-carotene.
Studies have shown that consuming 20 cherries per day may be as effective as aspirin at relieving pain [34].

Tart cherries in particular have been described as having one of the highest concentrations of anti-oxidants. They contain high levels of **anthocyanins** which significantly reduce muscle pain and improve joint pain [35].

A pilot study carried out by the Baylor Research Institute in 2007 tested the benefits of cherries in helping to alleviate the symptoms of OA. They found that over half the number of patients given cherry pills for 8 weeks reported improvements in joint function and less pain. *(the cherry pills were made up from ground montmorency cherries in a soft gelatin capsule) [36].

Other studies have also suggested that cherries could be effective in reducing the symptoms of osteoarthritis (OA). Patients with inflammatory OA who drank two 10.5-ounce bottles of tart cherry juice daily resulted in a significant reduction in inflammatory markers [37].

Larger trials are needed to be carried out to confirm the effect of cherries on OA. But due to the high anti-oxidant levels in cherries and these promising findings, eating a bunch of cherries or drinking a glass of cherry juice could be beneficial to OA sufferers.

4. Dark Chocolate

Dark chocolate is rich in flavonoids – which is an anti-oxidant.

Try eating one small square - 2-3 times per week. Recommended amounts are 50g per week.

Dark chocolate must have a minimum of 70% cocoa solids [38].

5. Garlic

It contains a compound called **diallyl disulphide** which lowers the level of enzymes which cause cartilage to breakdown.

A study assessed the food intake of over 1000 pairs of healthy twins. The study found that diets which were high in fruit and vegetables had a beneficial effect in preventing the onset of early signs of hip OA. *Non citrus fruits and alliums (onions, leeks and in particular **garlic**) had the most protective effect [39].

6. Ginger

Ginger is a tropical plant with an aromatic stem (called a rhizome) which grows underground. It contains active components that stop the body from producing inflammatory substances that affect the joints. Ginger works by interfering and reducing the production of prostaglandins and leukotriene which are both inflammatory compounds.

It has been reported that using ginger regularly helps reduce the pain and swelling in joints due to its strong anti-inflammatory effect [40].

There are many ways to include ginger in your diet and can be used fresh or dried as a spice:

-Grated or sliced ginger can be used in marinades, stir fries and curries.

-Add thin slices of ginger when grilling or steaming veggies, fish and meats.

-Use fresh or powdered ginger in fruit crumbles and stewed or baked fruits.

-You can use fresh ginger to make a tea by pouring boiling water over sliced or grated ginger. (use honey to sweeten the tea if required).

7. Green Tea

This tea contains powerful antioxidants called **catechins** which neutralise free radicals [41]. Studies by researchers at the University of Sheffield have discovered even more benefits of drinking catechin rich green tea – specifically the catchetins EPCG (epigallocatechin gallate) and ECG (epicatechin gallate).

These catechins can block enzymes that destroy cartilage – reducing pain/swelling in the joints. Drinking green tea should be seen as taking a preventative measure in the damage of cartilage [42].

If you are taking green tea extract, aim for 250mg to 500mg daily---or drink a couple of cups of green tea daily. 2 - 3 cups of green tea per day are recommended (for a total of 240 - 320 mg polyphenols) or 100 - 750 mg per day of standardized green tea extract is recommended. Caffeine-free versions are available and recommended [43].

8. Good Fats

There are good fats which are anti-inflammatory and essential to include in your diet. They provide the building blocks for cells and hormones which are essential to ensure the proper functioning of all our body systems. This includes healing tissues and producing the lubricating fluid in our joints.

Healthy fats contain monounsaturated or omega-3 fats.Commonly used vegetable oils such as sunflower, corn and safflower oils are high in polyunsaturated fats and omega 6 fats. They are often genetically modified. Cooking with these oils creates harmful toxins and trans fats as a result of oxidation processes through being heated. Choose fats rich in monounsaturated fats (olive oil) and omega-3s and low in omega-6 fatty acids.

Healthy choices: coconut, olive, avocado, nut and seed oils - including hemp and flaxseeds

Coconut oil

Coconut oil has been cited as one of the best anti-inflammatory fats. It contains lauric acid which has both anti-oxidant and anti-microbial properties. A large percentage of coconut oil is made up of saturated fatty acids. This has given coconut oil a bad press because saturated fats have been linked with the development of cardio vascular disease. An analysis of studies has shown that there is no clear link [44].

The type of saturated fat in coconut oil is a natural unprocessed plant-based fat. Plus the majority of the fatty acids in coconut oil are made up of medium –chain triglycerides (MCT's). In comparison, most vegetable oils are made up of long chain triglycerides (LCT's). LCT's are larger molecules which your body finds harder to break down so it is easier to store them as fat [45].

MCT's are smaller so they can be digested quickly and are then burned straight away by our liver to create energy. Therefore, our body uses this fat source for energy rather than storing it up. Coconut oil increases our metabolism and does not raise insulin levels quickly [46].

Always use unrefined, cold-pressed coconut oil. Coconut oil is great to use in cooking and can replace oils and butters either during cooking processes like stir-frying or baking or to add to cooked veggies, as a spread on bread/toast or in your bowl of morning porridge.

Extra-virgin Olive Oil

This oil contains a compound called oleocanthal, which prevents the production of pro-inflammatory enzymes (COX -1 and CO-2) in the same way that NSAIDs do.

Researchers found the intensity of the "peppery flavour or bite" in olive oil is directly related to the amount of oleocanthal it contains.
The stronger-flavored extra virgin olive oils contain the highest levels of oleocanthal [47].

Avocado Oil

It is rich in monounsaturated fats and has been shown to boost levels of good cholesterol HDL, while lowering C-reactive protein, a marker of inflammation in the blood [48].
Try avocado oil as an alternative to olive oil in salad dressings or as a dip for breads.

*Monounsaturated olive and avocado oils should only be used in small quantities as they can promote inflammation when eaten in large amounts).

Grapeseed oil:

It is extracted from the seeds of grapes. It is rich in vitamin E and oleic acid, an omega-9 fatty acid that may help reduce food cravings. Grapeseed oil has a high smoke point which makes it great to use for cooking [48].

Walnut oil:

It contains 10 times more omega-3 fatty acids than olive oil. To preserve its health benefits and great taste, do not heat this oil [48].

Flax seed oil :

It is a good source of Omega 3 – but not to be used for cooking [48].

Limit your Intake

It is still wise to use oil in small amounts. Remember they are high in calories (one tbsp. contains over 100 calories [49].

9. Herbs and Spices

Spices contain lots of nutrients which have anti-inflammatory effects and they add great flavour to food. Spices add wonderful flavour and have loads of health benefits. Use these herbs and spices generously to pack flavour into foods. In particular, turmeric and ginger are powerful, natural anti-inflammatory agents [50].

Beneficial Herbs and Spices:

- Turmeric

- Ginger

- Rosemary

- Basil

- Chives

- Sage

- Thyme

- Oregano

- Parsley

- Black Pepper

- Cardamom

- Cloves

- Chilli

- Cayenne Pepper

- Cinnamon

- Coriander

10. Strawberries

Strawberries contain **phenols** which reduce the activity of cyclooxygenase (COX) enzymes.

Phenols may lower blood levels of C-reactive protein (CRP), an inflammatory marker according to researchers at the Harvard School of Public Health [51].

Fresh or frozen strawberries are recommended.

11. Turmeric

It contains the active ingredient **curcumin** which is an anti-inflammatory and a powerful antioxidant. It lowers two enzymes which cause inflammation [52].

Studies have shown that curcumin may be effective at reducing the pain and inflammation caused by OA. A study using a supplement combining turmeric, ginger and boswellia was found to may help relieve symptoms in knee OA [53].

Another study found that patients who took turmeric supplements for 90 days, reported a 58% reduction in pain and were able to reduce their painkillers. Blood tests showed lower levels of C-reactive protein (an inflammatory compound) [54].

*Important note - studies have found that curcumin has poor bioavailability. This means that it is not absorbed easily into the body because it is broken down too quickly in the intestines and liver [55].

In order to help absorb it better, it has been recommended to take curcumin combined with **piperine,** extracted from black pepper,which enhances the absorption of curcumin. Therefore always remember to use black pepper along with turmeric in your recipes.

Other Beneficial Vitamins

Vitamin B3 (niacinamide):

A few studies have shown that vitamin B3 can improve symptoms of osteoarthritis by improving joint flexibility and reducing inflammation. It may even be able to reduce the amount of pain-killers needed to ease symptoms [56].

It plays many roles in the body and is needed for maintaining healthy cells. Although researchers aren't exactly sure why, a diet high in niacin may help protect people from developing osteoarthritis in the first place. Some studies show that niacin may cut the risk of developing osteoarthritis risk by half [57].

Vitamin B3 is found in yeast, meat, fish, milk, eggs, green vegetables, and cereal grains [58].

Excellent food sources:

shitake mushrooms and tuna.

Very good sources include:

salmon, chicken breast, asparagus, halibut and venison [59].

Vitamin D

Vitamin D not only helps prevent the breakdown of cartilage, it's necessary for rebuilding healthy cartilage and maintaining strong bones. A large percentage of OA sufferers have been found to have lower levels of vitamin D. Vitamin D deficiency is also associated with inflammation. A low vitamin D has also been linked to osteoarthritis directly [60].

Increasing vitamin D levels improve muscle strength and improve joint function. By getting plenty of vitamin D in your diet, joint damage progresses more slowly. A lack of vitamin causes joint damage to develop very quickly, leading to significant joint disability [61].

Vitamin D rich foods include salmon, sardines, tuna, prawns, liver and dairy products. To address their higher risk for D deficiency, the elderly population are encouraged to take a vitamin D supplement of 400-600 IU per day.

It is recommended to take 600 IU per day after the age 60.

Caution

Vitamin D can be toxic in high doses so you must not exceed recommended doses [62].

Water

Water is needed to eliminate waste i.e toxins. If you are dehydrated, waste products are not eliminated and they get stored in the body. Aim to drink 2 litres throughout day. If this is not part of your regular routine, introduce water into your day gradually.

Try managing 2-3 glasses per day and build up. Or keep a bottle with you that you can sip from regularly. If you struggle with the lack of flavour, try making drinks that are made of mostly water (herbal teas, highly diluted fruit juice, water with lemon, lime or orange slices)

In a Nutshell

There are a wide variety of foods that are anti-inflammatory and have the power to fight diseases and illnesses. These foods are packed with a variety of nutrients which can prevent oxidative stress or inhibit inflammatory pathways that are responsible for creating chronic inflammation. Make sure your diet is rich in omega 3's, healthy fats, fruits, vegetables, wholegrains, nuts, seeds, herbs and spices.

11. Step 3 - Balance Blood Sugar Levels

Quick rises in blood sugars create biochemical changes in cells which are pro-inflammatory. Reducing sugary and high-glycemic foods is a really important way to decrease inflammation. Keeping your blood sugars levels balanced keeps your body working at its best. You can maintain a good balance by eating regular small meals, limiting sugar and refined carbs and eating more protein.

Insulin is released whenever your blood sugar level is raised. Eating sugars and refined carbohydrates create large spikes of insulin. Low glycemic foods release their sugar content slowly into the blood stream and prevent sudden spikes in insulin levels which promote inflammation.

High and Low Glycemic Foods

Foods with **higher glycemic loads** affect inflammation by raising an inflammatory compound called CRP (*C-reactive protein*) which is damaging to joints. Long-term consumption of foods with a high glycemic load also appears to be linked to a greater risk to obesity, diabetes, and inflammation [63].

The Glycemic Load (GL) of a food is the amount of carbohydrate that is easily broken down into simple sugars.

The Glycemic Index (GI) is a measure of the degree to which a carbohydrate is likely to raise your blood sugar (glucose) levels. The scale runs from 0 to 100 (with 0 being low and 100 being high).

The higher the **GL** of a food is, the greater the rise in blood sugar levels. Higher blood sugar levels increase insulin levels and increase levels of inflammation.

Foods with a **GL of 10** or below are classed as low.

Foods with a **GL of 20** or above increase levels of inflammation and increase the risk of joint damage [64].

Keep your insulin levels down

- Combine carbs with fat or protein: nuts with dried fruit, fresh fruit with a piece of cheese or spread with nut butters, mashed avocado (add a splash of lemon juice or sliced boiled egg on wholegrain toast

- Add acid: marinate meat and veggies with lemon or lime juice . Use vinegars or lemon/lime juice in salad dressings.

- Cook your pasta so it is still slightly firm (al dente) as this reduces its glycemic load [65].

In a Nutshell

If your diet is high in refined carbohydrates and high glycemic foods it will raise your blood sugar levels. It takes longer for your body to breakdown foods with a lower glycemix index. This means that it takes longer to break them down into sugars, which is then released more slowly into your blood stream avoiding those quick spikes in blood sugar levels.   High blood sugar levels are associated with high levels of inflammation. Keeping your blood sugars balanced by eating lower glycemic foods help reduce inflammation.

12. Step 4 - Eliminate anti-arthritic foods

You have learned about pro-inflammatory foods which trigger inflammatory pathways in the body and these should be avoided. These foods include processed foods, trans fats, high glycemic foods, foods rich in omega 6's and arachidonic acid and synthetic substances such as sweeteners, additives and preservatives. Some of you may notice a significant improvement in your symptoms by greatly reducing or eliminating these foods from your diet. A certain percentage of individuals can also suffer from their own specific set of food intolerances.

Elimination Diets

Intolerances and sensitivities to foods create inflammation so removing these foods from your diet that you are makes sense. An elimination diet can help figure out if you are sensitive or intolerant to certain foods that could be contributing to your symptoms. You will learn how your body responds to different foods.

An elimination diet is where you remove certain foods from your diet for a specific period of time. After that time is up, the eliminated food is slowly reintroduced while you monitor yourself for symptoms

The key is to keep track of your symptoms in a diary during to get a clear picture of what has happened to your symptoms.

How Do They Work?

Give up a food type/group for 3 weeks. Common food groups to create intolerances and sensitivities include:

- Dairy products

- Citrus Fruits

- Wheat

- Gluten/Lectins (wheat, rye, oats, legumes, pulses)

- All sugar apart from fruits

- Nightshade vegetables (*some people need to remove nightshade foods for a longer time than 3 weeks to see results)

- Soy products

Some people remove all these food groups during an elimination diet. Hypoallergenic foods that you can eat during such a strict elimination phase include lamb, turkey, fish, rice, most fruits and vegetables (apart from citrus and nightshades if you are testing them). It is up to you to decide how many food groups and which ones you would like to remove.

If you feel you may be sensitive to other foods, eliminate them for 3 weeks i.e. coffee/black tea, chocolate, meat etc.

You will be more successful if you find recipes using foods you can eat in advance. Making some dishes and snacks in advance is really useful as you can quickly satisfy any hunger pangs without straying off the diet.

Note how you feel during the elimination period. Record your notes in the morning, afternoon and evening.

At the end of the 3 week period, you will add one food category back at a time into your diet and see which ones affect your symptoms.

Re-introduction

At the end of the 3 weeks of elimination, reintroduce one food group throughout that day. Record any symptoms or reactions for the following 2 days after the day you reintroduced that food.

If you have no symptoms after those 2 days, you can reintroduce another food the next day (the day after the 2 days you have monitored yourself for symptoms). You can continue this pattern of, reintroducing one new food every few days, until you've identified if any foods are causing any problems. ***Re-introduce the food 2-3 times during the day**

Dairy Elimination

Have some yogurt in the morning, some cheese at lunch and a glass of milk in the evening. Record everything you eat that day. Notice how you feel within a period of 3-4 hours after you have eaten dairy. Record your symptoms (if you feel well –write "no symptoms").

Nightshade Elimination

Give up white potatoes, tomatoes, peppers, chillies and aubergines for 3 weeks and observe your symptoms. You can substitute sweet potatoes for potatoes during this time. After the 3 weeks are up, add one type of nightshade every 3 days. Only test one nightshade food at a time – so if you started introducing tomatoes on the first day after the elimination don't eat other nightshades. Keep notes of any changes to your symptoms as you reintroduce each one back to your diet.

For example:

Day 1 (after elimination) – eat tomatoes or drink tomato juice 2- 3 times that day. Don't forget to record symptoms after a few hours. Observe if any of the eliminated nightshades trigger any of your symptoms on that day. If it does, you are sensitive to that vegetable. You should reduce or eliminate it from your diet.

*If no symptoms occur on the test day or 2 days after, that food is safe. If a food causes symptoms, you are sensitive to it and must eliminate or greatly reduce it from your diet [66, 67, 68].

In a Nutshell

Elimination diets can be useful if you suspect that a certain food or food group could be responsible for flaring up your symptoms. An elimination diet is done by removing a certain food or foods for a set period of time while you monitor your symptoms. Common food groups implicated in triggering symptoms of OA include dairy, gluten/wheat, sugars, citrus fruits, nightshades and soy. It may be useful to consult a medical practitioner before you start an elimination diet.

13. Step 5 - Add herbs and supplements that reduce joint inflammation and support cartilage

In addition to an excellent diet, natural herbals or supplements can be a key part of your plan to overcome acute or chronic pain. Anti-inflammatory medications can be harmful to the stomach, and in addition cause risky side effects.

You should, however, seek your doctor's advice when taking any supplements if you have any underlying medical conditions, to avoid any complications with medications you are already taking or to prevent an allergic reaction.

What are Dietary Supplements?

Dietary supplements include vitamins, minerals and botanicals.

Dietary supplements are not classed as drugs, but they can still act like medication. They are intended to be taken in addition to a healthy diet. They are not a replacement for a healthy diet. Talk to your doctor about any supplements you are considering using.

Plants produce chemicals that can have effects on the body ranging from mild to potent, just like the chemicals in your medication. They **can** interact and interfere with medication.

If you have any medical conditions, certain supplements can be dangerous to take. **That's why you need to get approval from your doctor about any supplement you are considering taking.**

Remember…..

Always tell your doctor if you are taking supplements or if you are thinking about taking a supplement while you are on medication or if have any medical conditions. A supplement may lead to overmedication and can interact negatively, which can have serious side effects. Never stop taking any prescribed medications while you are trying a supplement before discussing this with your doctor. It may not be safe to stop your medical treatment and rely on supplements alone.

It is always important to carry out your own research for any supplement you are interested in taking.

Checklist to go through before taking a supplement

- Are there clinical studies to show the supplement is effective?

- Is this supplement safe to use?

- Are there any potential side effects?

- What is the recommended dose?

- How often should you take it?

- Should it be taken with food?

- Will it interact with or affect any medications you are on?

- Will it aggravate any medical conditions you have?

- Will it interact negatively with any other supplements you are taking?

- How long before you should see any results?

Things to do once you have started taking a supplement

- Try one new supplement at a time

- Keep a record of its effects

- Let your doctor know which supplements you are taking

- Keep a list of all of the supplements you are taking

Never take more than the recommended amount as overdosing on supplements can be as dangerous as overdosing on medication.

* If you experience any unusual symptoms or feel worse after using a supplement, call your doctor as soon as possible. It is handy to keep the bottle the supplement came in so that you can show your doctor.

Phytodolor

A herbal supplement which contains aspen leaf, golden rod herb and common ash bark extract. It is sold in the form of a tincture and is known as STW1. This mixture of herbs provides anti-oxidant, anti-inflammatory and analgesic (pain reducing) effects as they contain a combination of salicyns, phenolic acids and quercetin.

Beneficial Effects:

Effective and safe pain relief which allows users to reduce the use of NSAID's and painkillers [69].

Studies:

There have been over 40 studies which have tested the effects of phytodolor for arthritis symptoms. So far most of the studies have reported positive results with significant improvements seen as soon as 3 days in some individuals but it can take up to 4 weeks to see results [70].

Effectiveness:

A review carried out by the Arthritis Research Campagin to assess the effectiveness of various supplements (ARC) found phytolodor to have a good level of effectiveness giving it a 4 points out of a possible 5 for effectiveness [71].

Dosage:

20-40 drops taken in water/ juice 3-4 times a day.

Side Effects:

Phytodolor is said to be safe with minimal side effects.

Interactions with Medication:

No known interactions with medications.

Contra-Indications:

Individuals with liver disease, gastric/duodenal ulcers epilepsy and pregnant/breastfeeding women [72].

SAMe: S-adenosylmethionine

SAM-e is a natural substance found in the cells of your body.

Beneficial Effects:

It helps to reduce joint pain, stiffness and swelling while improving mobility and rebuilding cartilage. SAM-e works as an anti-inflammatory and pain-reliever for osteoarthritic joints. If effective for you, results are quick with relief occurring within a week [73].

Studies:

Many studies have established that SAMe has effective anti-inflammatory and pain relieving properties in the treatment of osteoarthritis. It is said to reduce pain as effectively as NSAID's with minimal side effects. Studies have also shown it stimulates the production of collagen and proteoglycans (which are components of cartilage) [74].

Effectiveness:

It is likely effective. The ARC review gave SAM-e a rating of 4points out of 5 for effectiveness [71].

Dosage:

400 – 1,200 mg daily [75].

Side effects:

Nausea, flatulence, diarrhea, dry mouth and headaches rarely occur and are mild in nature.

Interactions with Medication:

SAM-e can increase risk of bleeding so is not advised to be used if you are taking blood thinners. It can increase the action of anti-depressant medications so it is not recommended to take it if you are on these meds.

Contra-indications:

It use is contra-indicated in people suffering from depression, bipolar disorder and Parkinson's disease [76].

Rosehip Powder

Rosehip powder is extracted from the wild rose- *rosa canina*. The extract comes from the red fruit that ripens when the flower dies. Rosehips contain polyphenols and anthocyanins which are anti-inflammatory and also have a high concentration of vitamin C [77].

Beneficial Effects:

Has consistent anti-inflammatory and anti-oxidative properties and significantly reduces joint pain. Patients on rosehip powder were less likely to use other pain medications

Studies:

Studies and analyses of clinical trials have found that treatment with rosehip powder has been shown to be consistent in reducing pain in arthritic patients. In contrast to nonsteroidal anti-inflammatory drugs and aspirin, rosehip has anti- inflammatory effects without the side-effects [78].

Patients with hip or knee OA were randomly given either 2.5 g of rosehip powder or placebo twice a day for 4 months. Results found that rosehip powder significantly reduced pain and improved hip flexion [79].

Rosehip powder was given to patients with OA of the knee, hip and hand. Results showed that 82% of these patients reported a significant improvement in pain reduction after three months [80]. Treatment with rosehip powder consistently reduced pain scores and that patients were twice as likely to respond to rosehip as compared to a placebo [81].

Effectiveness:

There is good evidence for the effectiveness of rosehip powder to reduce pain in osteoarthritic patients The ARC review gave it a 3 out 5 [71].

Side effects:

Mild constipation, diarrhoea and heartburn.

Interactions with Medications:

Can increase the effects of oestrogen in oestrogen-based medications. It can also interact negatively with blood thinners (aspirin and warfarin) and lithium [82].

Contra-Indications:

Not advised if you suffer from blood disorders such as thalassemia, sideroblastic anemia, sickle cell anemia, hemochromatosis and glucose-6 phosphate dehydrogenase deficiency. May not be safe if you are pregnant or breastfeeding [83].

Avocado-Soybean Unsaponifiables (ASU's)

This is a supplement made up of one-third of avocado oil and two-thirds of soybean oil.

Beneficial Effects:

ASU's have good anti-inflammatory effects and have been shown to reduce a variety of inflammatory compounds. ASU's also prevent the destruction of cartilage caused by inflammatory chemicals called interleukins. They also aids in cartilage repair by stimulating the production of collagen [84].

Studies:

Studies have shown beneficial effects in taking ASU's in patients suffering from knee and hip OA [85]. It can take 3 months of taking this supplement before any results can be seen.

Effectiveness:

There is good evidence for the effectiveness of ASU's in reducing symptoms in knee and hip OA . A review (in which 4 trials and one review were evaluated) concluded that there is good evidence for taking ASU's for relieving symptoms of OA but further studies recommended to investigate long-term effects are needed [86].

Dosage:

300 mg of ASU for three months is effective in reducing pain and inflammation [87].

Side Effects:

Most commonly reported side-effects include allergic reactions and stomach upset [88].

Interactions with Medication

May increase your risk of bleeding if you are taking blood thinners such as aspirin, heparin and warfarin. ASU's can significantly raise your blood pressure if you take them with anti-depressant drugs called monoamine oxidase inhibitors (MAOIs).

Contra-Indications:

You shouldn't take ASU if have allergies to latex, bananas, peaches and chestnuts as this increases the risk of having an allergic reaction [89].

Pine Bark Extract (Pycnogenol)

A plant extract from the bark of the French maritime pine tree with anti-oxidant properties

Beneficial Effects:

It can reduce the pain and stiffness in OA sufferers, in particular those suffering from knee OA [90].

Studies:

A study of 156 patients with knee osteoarthritis received 100 milligrams of Pycnogenol for three months. Results demonstrated that over half of patients experienced a reduction in their symptoms (56%) and could reduce the use of their pain medications (58%) [91].

Effectiveness:

Results have demonstrated that pine bark provided pain relief and is an effective treatment for osteoarthritis symptoms however more evidence is needed to rate pycnogenol for these uses. The ARC only gave it a rating of 2 out 5 for effectiveness [71].

Dosage:

Not currently established but studies have used 2 tablets containing 50 mg.

Side Effects:

Dizziness, headaches, mouth ulcers and stomach upsets.

Interactions with Medications:

Cholesterol, blood pressure, blood-thinning or diabetic medications, immunosuppressants or NSAID's. It may interfere with some chemotherapy drugs due to its anti-oxidant content.

Contra-indications:

Do not use if pregnant or breastfeeding. It may lower blood sugar levels so be cautious if you are diabetic or hypoglycemic [92].

Glucosamine Sulphate

It is an important structural protein which is a major component of joint cartilage. It is derived from the shells of shellfish.

Beneficial Effects:

It helps to repair cartilage. Glucosamine can also help rebuild both cartilage and synovial fluid. In some studies it produced consistent benefits such as improved joint range of movement while protecting the joint from further damage.

Studies:

Glucosamine has been shown to be effective in some studies in relieving joint pain and inflammation in sufferers of knee osteoarthritis

One study showed that glucosamine may reduce the risk of osteoarthritis progression by 54% using a 1500mg dose daily [93].

A four week study (using over 170 patients with osteoarthritis of the knee) compared the effects of glucosamine sulphate at a dose of 1500 mg/day compared to 1200 mg/day of ibuprofen. Glucosamine relieved the symptoms as effectively as ibuprofen. Less side effects were reported by the group taking glucosamine than the group taking ibuprofen [94].

Another study showed that participants with moderate-to-severe hip or knee osteoarthritis (receiving 1,500 mg of glucosamine combined with 200 mg of omega-3) had greater pain reduction and fewer symptoms than those who took glucosamine by itself [95].

Glucosamine is as effective as NSAIDs for easing osteoarthritic symptoms but may take twice as long to start working [96].

Effectiveness:

There have been many trials conducted to study the effectiveness of glucosamine. Results are mixed as trial results are varied, leading to conflicting views in its effectiveness. The ARC review gave glucosamine sulfate a score of 2 out 5 for effectiveness [71].

Dosage:

1000-1500 mg daily

Side Effects:

Glucosamine can cause mild stomach upsets, nausea, diarrhoea and heartburn.

Interactions with Medication:

Can interfere with diabetes medication, cholesterol or blood pressure medicines.

Contraindications:

Consult your doctor before taking glucosamine if you have diabetes or suffer from glucose tolerance. It is unclear if glucosamine can increase insulin resistance in humans.

*Note: Glucosamine is derived from shellfish so check with your GP if you are allergic to shellfish

Chondroitin Sulphate

Chondroitin sulphate is a structural component of cartilage. It works by stimulating cartilage production, while preventing enzymes and free radicals from destroying it. It also improves circulation to inflamed joints which allows antioxidants and glucosamine to enter and begin the repair process.

Beneficial Effects:

Reduce pain and inflammation while improving joint function and slowing down the progression of arthritis. Some sufferers taking chondroitin are able to decrease their use of NSAID's [97].

Studies:

A few studies have shown very good results from long-term treatment with chondroitin sulphate.

One study investigated the effects of prescribing 800 mg of chondroitin sulphate to a group of people with osteoarthritis for over 3 years. The results indicated that the chondroitin sulphate significantly reduced pain, and increased joint mobility. In addition, the joints were protected from further progression of osteoarthritis [98].

A large NIH trial of glucosamine and chondroitin showed that the supplements are more effective for decreasing pain when combined than alone in patients with moderate to severe symptoms. Due to the smaller number of participants in this group, they highlighted the need for further studies to evaluate its effectiveness [99].

Effectiveness:

Possibly effective, results from trials have been mixed with the ARC giving it a low rating of 2 out of 5 for effectiveness [71].

Dosage:

800 mg to 1,200 mg daily in two to four divided doses. Often combined with glucosamine. Allow up to one month to notice effect.

Side Effects:

Stomach upsets, nausea and diarrhoea.

Interactions with Medication:

Consult your doctor before taking chondroitin if you are taking warfarin or if you suffer from hemophilia. Chondroitin can have blood thinning activity.

Contra-indications: Not to be taken if you are pregnant or breastfeeding, asthmatic or suffering from prostate cancer (or if it runs in your family –brother/father) [100].

Methylsulfonylmethane – MSM

MSM is an organic sulfur compound. Sulfur is needed to form connective tissue.

Beneficial Effects:

It reduces pain and inflammation by acting as an analgesic by reducing nerve impulses that transmit pain to the brain.

Studies:

Studies have indicated that arthritic joints have a lower sulphur content. A 2006 pilot study of 50 men and women with knee osteoarthritis showed that 6,000 mg of MSM improved symptoms of pain and physical function without major side effects [101].

Effectiveness:

MSM was rated 2 out of 5 for effectiveness by the ARC review [71].

Dosage:

1,000 mg to 3,000 mg daily to be taken with food

Side Effects:

Can cause stomach upset or diarrhea.

Interactions with Medication:

Do not use if you are taking blood thinners.

Contra-Indications:

Safety when pregnant or breast-feeding not known [102].

In a Nutshell

There are a lot of supplements out there which are recommended to manage the symptoms of OA, to support joint cartilage repair and/or to reduce the rate of cartilage destruction. Some of these supplements are backed by good scientific evidence. It is very important to research claims that are made regarding the benefits of a particular supplement. Always be aware of any side effects and risks associated with any particular supplement. Always check with your doctor before starting a supplement as they can interfere with certain medications and are not

recommended if you suffer from certain medical conditions.

14. Other Factors and Lifestyle Changes

Cooking techniques

High Cooking Temperatures

Frying or grilling certain foods at high temperatures produces compounds that can increase inflammation in the body.

The compounds are known as **AGES -advanced glycation end products.** These free radical scavengers are found in the blood of people with diseases associated with inflammation, including osteoarthritis.

Fight the AGES - Keeping it healthy

Turn down the heat

High cooking temperatures create chemical reactions from sugars and proteins reacting in the heat that can produce toxic compounds such as AGE's which can damage DNA. Cooking with higher and dryer heat causes more AGEs to form. Meats particularly those higher in fat produce the highest levels of AGE's. So swap frying, grilling, roasting or barbecuing for steaming, poaching, stewing and braising [103].

Marinate your meat

The formation of AGEs can be greatly minimized by using acidic ingredients like lemon or vinegar. The acid lowers the pH level of what you are cooking in turn slowing glycation, The amount of AGE's were reduced by half after being marinated for an hour [104].

So go and research different marinade recipes for your meat if you do decide to grill, fry or roast. It is not only delicious but protects you from the effect of AGE's.

Cooking with Oils

The smoke point of an oil is the temperature that it needs to reach for a vapour (smoke) to develop. This is the point when the oil starts to breakdown causing chemical changes which produces harmful toxins such free radicals. Certain oils and fats are able to be heated at higher temperatures without changing their chemical composition.

Saturated fats are healthier to cook with, as they are more stable when heated whereas polyunsaturated fats are not. Plant-based saturated fats include coconut and palm oil. Animal-based saturated fats include butter and lard.

Even choosing butter on occasions (in small quantities) to cook with, is a better option than using polyunsaturated oils (sunflower, corn, rapeseed (canola) and safflower oils).

High quality extra virgin olive oil can be used as it is a monounsaturated fat which is also more stable than polyunsaturated oils when heated.

Tips for reducing AGES:

It is very important to lower the cooking temperature of fish and meats [103].

- Reduce the amount of grilled, roasted, fried and microwaved meats in your diet.

- Steam fish and seafood.

- Poach, simmer, stew or braise meats in sauces or stock.

- Reduce your intake of processed foods as they are usually cooked at high temperatures to prolong their shelf life

Benefits of Exercise

In order for any nutritional program to work effectively, it must be combined with exercise. This could be part of the reason why some studies looking at the effects of nutrients and supplements in reducing symptoms of arthritis do not show stronger evidence.

Joints require motion to stay healthy. Being inactive not only causes stiffness in your joints but causes the associated muscles and soft tissues around the joints to weaken and waste away. Osteoarthritis affects the normal alignment of the joint which leads to muscle weakness and imbalances.

A painful arthritic joint stops you from using it so you walk less and give up on exercise.

The muscles around the arthritic joint get weaker which puts more strain on the joint itself. The lack of movement and exercise can lead to weight gain which causes even more stress on your joints.

Regular exercise can prevent joints from stiffening up as well as stimulating circulation and healing. Exercise also improves joint flexibility, strength and balance. Osteoarthritis sufferers who exercise regularly generally suffer from less pain and can get on with their daily activities including household chores and hobbies.

Exercise also leads to weight loss, which is important for people with osteoarthritis.

Incorporating Exercise

Exercise and movement are essential in any joint health management program.

To make the most of the vital nutrients you are eating to support your joints - you also need to make sure these nutrients are getting delivered to the joint and cartilage.

The only way to do this properly is through movement. The cartilage in joints depends on movement of the joint so that it can absorb nutrients directly from joint fluid – motion is lotion. It is extremely difficult for nutrients to get to the cartilage when there is minimal or no movement in the joint.

Your exercise program should consist of a combination of low-impact aerobics, strength training (including core strengthening) and stretching. You should always check with your doctor before starting any exercise program.

Cardiovascular (Aerobic) Exercise

Cardiovascular or aerobic exercise provides a good workout for the heart and lungs while burning lots of calories. It is recommended to take part in low impact cardiovascular exercise which still provides a good aerobic workout with minimal stress on the joints. Benefits of aerobic exercise include weight loss, keeping your heart healthy and help to keep joints stable and flexible. Low impact workouts include:

- Walking

- Swimming

- Cross-trainer (elliptical machine)

- Water Aerobics

- Cycling

Exercising in water is highly recommended for people with arthritis. Arthritic patients should avoid high-impact sports, such as jogging, tennis, squash and racquetball.

Strengthening Exercises

The National Institute for Clinical Excellence (NICE) recommends including exercise which helps to strengthen muscles. This includes weight training and isometrics. Strength training is needed to balance aerobic exercise. To improve muscle strength and control it there needs to be repeated muscle activity with greater resistance than your normal daily activities.

Isometric exercise is a type of resistance strength training. Isometrics are done by pushing or pulling against an immovable object or by holding the muscle in a fixed position for a set period of time. The muscle is contracted but its length does not change and there is no movement at the joint. Isometrics exercises can be used for general muscle conditioning but they are also appropriate for rehabilitation where you can strengthen your muscles without placing stress on your joints. They increase muscle strength while burning fat and maintaining bone density.

Core Strengthening

To increase muscle strength in the torso, the core body muscles (abs and back muscles) need to be specifically targeted.

Flexibility and Conditioning Exercises:

Good examples are pilates, yoga, Tai-chi and Qui Gong as they build strength particularly in the core muscles and are gentle on the joints. They also incorporate stretching and slightly elevate your heart rate. They focus on maintaining flexibility, strength, balance and proper breathing which help to control arthritic pain. They also have an effect on mental wellness by improving your overall well-being and reducing feelings of anxiety. Other great benefits are that they help to lower stress levels and reduce blood pressure.

Recommendations:

20 to 30 minutes a day of aerobic exercise (5-7 week) is recommended. 5-10 minutes of stretching (before and after exercising is important. Strengthening exercises should be limited to every other day to allow muscles to recover. It is important to develop an exercise routine that is realistic for you to achieve. If you are new to exercising, you can build it up gradually with 2-3 exercise sessions per week. Walk to your local shop or go for 20-30 min walk around the block to build in your 5-7 aerobic sessions – it doesn't all have to be in the gym.

Physical Therapy

For people suffering with arthritis, physical therapy such as chiropractic, physiotherapy or massage may be needed to improve joint strength and flexibility before you start an exercise routine. In addition to exercise, manipulation of muscles and joints by a trained therapist can be a great combination to reduce your symptoms.

In a Nutshell

Light to moderate exercise has been shown to help prevent the onset of osteoarthritis. Exercise is important to increase muscle strength and tone around your joints. Exercise is beneficial because it can improve the health of affected joints as it can enhance its repair capacity. Exercise improves the circulation around the joint which helps to reduce pain and stiffness. It also strengthens the muscles around joints which improves its shock absorbency capability.

15. Putting It All Together

Eating healthy is not about living on lettuce and celery sticks. There is a wide range of exciting, flavourful foods that can help load up with nutrients that nourish your joints.

The best way to protect your joints is to eat a wide variety of nutritious foods. You should design your meals around fresh fruits, vegetables, whole grains, legumes, fish, and lean meats.

So now that you have learned about the nutritional aspects of fighting the chronic inflammation … here is some help in applying all these principles into your daily eating routine. This process will involve time and hard work. You need to be invested and ready to take on the challenge.

If you are used to eating ready meals, processed food and take- aways, it can be really difficult to fight your cravings. If you are not used to cooking or don't really like cooking, it can be time-consuming to prepare fresh food. It does get quicker with practice.

The very first thing to incorporate into your diet is eating natural, unprocessed, nutrient packed foods.

Eat Clean

The first few weeks of your eating plan should focus on eliminating processed foods from your diet. Processed foods include: ready meals, smoked, cured, junk foods, sugar, refined carbohydrates, and foods loaded with additives and preservatives. Your body is able to rid itself of all the toxins that have accumulated in your body. Choose foods that are natural and free of chemicals, additives, preservatives and sweeteners.

Start adding more vegetables and fruits and wholegrains into your meals. Eat fish and grass fed, free range organic meats.

Experiment

Variety is the spice of life. You need to mix it up so that you don't get bored and go off your eating plan. Try different foods and see if you like them. Find recipes that appeal to you which using the recommended foods talked about in this book. You can research these recipes through the internet or books or ask friends. You will often come across dishes that you never would have thought of and absolutely love. It also makes the whole process a lot more fun. Make it delicious by picking vegetables, meats, fruits, nuts, oils, spices, to make meals thatfocus on quality and flavor.

Practice and Patience

It is very daunting to start eating clean or cooking up all these dishes if you are not a cook or don't enjoy cooking. If you are not used to cooking with fresh ingredients, it is time consuming to prepare everything. You will get faster as time goes on. If you really don't enjoy cooking, search the internet for quick, easy to prepare recipes

So over a period of time, you have a repertoire of recipes that you can prepare. It is also difficult to reduce foods that you love but are inflammatory. Don't beat yourself up if you have an off day or have a special event. Just get back on your eating plan and move forward.

Write it Down

Sticking to a food plan will work better if you write everything down. Keep a food journal and record what you eat daily to keep track of your progress.record of all the food that you eat and drink along with any symptoms you have experienced on a daily basis. Make sure you write down everything you eat and drink, including snacks. Aim to note down how you feel in the morning, afternoon and evening. See if you can notice any patterns where flare-ups of symptoms seem to be associated with any particular foods. You should feel more energised and healthy and may have even lost some weight.

Elimination Diet

Some of you may feel much better by just eating cleaner and don't need to test foods through an elimination diet. For others, arthritic symptoms can be triggered or worsened by a specific food or food group. Again it is very overwhelming and confusing to know how to eliminate foods as a lot of different people have different theories to what causes arthritis. Certain people claim that gluten and grains are blame while others recommend eliminating removing meat and dairy completely out of the diet for good. Certain foods like citrus fruits, nightshade vegetables are also worth checking as well.

This ebook is not a recipe book but I have written a section to give you a few ideas about how to start putting meals together. You can use these ideas as a starting point. Through this process, you will find recipes and foods that you love and over time you will develop an eating plan that works for you.

Breakfast Time

Ricotta or Greek yogurt

Sweeten your ricotta or yogurt using home-made stewed apple or cherries. Alternatively you can mash unsweetened dry figs or dates and mix in the ricotta or yogurt. Sprinkle with chopped nuts and seeds for a bit of crunch.

Toast

Use whole grain or seeded breads. Making your own bread is healthier.

Use coconut oil instead of butter.

Toast Toppings:

- nut butters (almond-cashew).

- mashed avocado with a squirt of lemon on it.

Oats/Porridge

Stir in a spoonful of unrefined coconut oil to your cooked porridge to make it creamy. Cook your porridge with almond or rice milk if you are reducing dairy.

Use a selection of healthy toppings to add flavour and texture

- Sprinkle seeds such as sunflower, pumpkin, flax, or linseed

- chopped nuts

- Add dried fruits – dried cranberries, blueberries, cherries or goji berries

- Add fresh fruit or berries,

Spices: cinnamon, nutmeg, ground ginger

Sweeten with a small amount of raw unpasteurized honey , agave nectar or maple syrup or unsweetened fruit compotes (stewed fruit) such as cherries, apples, pears .

Eggs

Instead of poaching, scrambling or boiling your eggs try an egg and veggie scramble

1. Fry your choice of chopped veggies until softened in a tbsp. of coconut or olive oil.

- courgettes (zucchini),

- artichoke hearts

- broccoli

- mushrooms (particularly shitake as they are packed with essential nutrients)

- spring onions, red onions

- peppers (bell) –(unless sensitive to nightshade)

- spinach

2. Add your choice of natural flavourings and soften for a couple more minutes:

- finely chopped garlic

- chopped herbs: thyme, parsley, chives, basil, oregano, rosemary

3. Then add organic or free range eggs and let it cook for a couple more minutes. Stir through occasionally if you want the egg to be more scrambled.

*Eggs go well with turmeric so this dish is a great way to get your intake of turmeric. Add a pinch of turmeric with a dash of black pepper while cooking your eggs.

4. Top with crumbled feta, grated fresh parmesan or cubed avocado with a dash of lemon.

Lunch and Dinner Ideas

Good lunches and dinners should consist of a portion of good protein and a load of veggies and unrefined carbohydrates.

Good Protein Choices

- good quality natural cheese and yogurt,

- omega-3 enriched, organic or free range eggs,

- free –range/organic poultry

- free-range /organic lean meats.

- fish

You should aim to reduce the amount of meat you eat. Buying organic or free –range cuts of meat are more expensive –but eating them fewer times per week becomes more cost-effective as well as being beneficial to our health.

Dairy - good options include goat's milk, greek yogurt, organic plain yogurt, ricotta cheese and hard cheeses such as emmental, jarlsberg, parmesan, edam, goat cheese and feta.

If you have a dairy intolerance or want to reduce the amount of dairy that you consume, try substituting cow's milk for rice or almond milk. Rice milk is hypo-allergenic.

Meat – choose leaner cuts of meats that are grass-fed or organic

Fish - various toxins are found in fish. The most harmful include mercury and pesticide residues and fish with highest levels of mercury are swordfish, kingfish, shark, marlin and tuna. You should reduce your consumption of these fish to once a week. Fish with lower levels of toxins include salmon, sardines and herrings.

Vegetables:

Eat more veggies: think of the rainbow and use all colours of veggies to get a good range of health-promoting phytonutrients.

Heavenly Hash

A hash is a filling way to get a good portion of healthy veggies in your meal. A veggie hash is made by using chopped up veggies which are then cooked in a pan with other ingredients like spices, onions/garlic and herbs.

- Use chopped up sweet potatoes, squash or brussel sprouts.

- Chop up sweet potatoes or squashes into cubes – it is best to parboil for 5 min or steam them for about 10 min. If using brussel sprouts, slice them up.

- Heat your oil (coconut/olive) in a large pan. If using onions, fry them on medium heat for 5 minutes until they have softened.

- Add the sweet potato, squash or sliced brussel sprouts to the pan. Press the veggies down with a spatula.

- Continue to let them cook for another 10-15 minutes, stirring a few times. The base of the veggies should form a browned crust.

- You can add spinach or steamed broccoli to the hash. Also remember to add your flavourings like fresh herbs or garlic.

Mega Mash

Use white beans such as cannellini or butter beans to make a mash. You can soften some finely chopped garlic in a tbsp. of olive oil and then add a tin of rinsed beans. Warm the beans through and mash them. Season the mash with a bit of sea salt, a splash of olive oil and lemon juice.

Stir fry Veggies

The combos are endless: pak choi, Chinese cabbage, spring greens, ribbons of carrots, strips of peppers, spring onions , mange- touts , baby corn, sugar snap peas,

shitake mushrooms. Add fresh grated ginger, chopped garlic and chilli flakes for a great flavour.

Soups

Soups are a great way to combine anti-oxidant rich vegetables with anti-inflammatory herbs and spices. Try carrot and ginger, butternut/pumpkin soups with turmeric and chilli.

Orange: use carrots, butternut squash or pumpkin for your soup. Use turmeric, curry powder, cayenne pepper, chili flakes or ginger to get the anti-inflammatory kick.

Carrot and ginger or butternut, turmeric, garlic and chilli are great combinations

Green: use a combination of green vegetables such as watercress, leeks, broccoli, spinach , spring greens. Use basil, thyme or parsley to add flavour.

Beans: Make broths with a combination of different beans, add celery, onions and carrot and green herbs such as thyme, parsley

Chicken: make Asian –style chicken broths using thin rice noodles. Use garlic, turmeric and ginger to increase anti-inflammatory effects

Salads

Vegetables and fruits: green leaves: romaine, little gem, spinach, rocket, watercress, chard, lambs lettuce.

Add your choice of tomatoes, peppers, cucumbers, grated carrot, red onions, spring onions, grated fresh beetroot, sugarsnap peas, radishes, raw broccoli florets, artichoke hearts, celery, corn, grated apple, slices of crisp pear, peas, green beans, asparagus

Protein: grated fresh parmesan, edam, feta cheese cube, goat's cheese , diced chicken breast, cold poached salmon fillet , mackerel, tuna, strips of steak. Or add beans such as chick peas.

Extra Flavour Punch: add shredded or chopped herbs - basil, mint, chives or thyme, parsley, tarragon, coriander. Chopped tarragon or basil goes with well with chicken or salmon.

Use homemade salad dressings –use extra virgin olive oil with an acid as a flavouring such as: lemon juice, lime, orange, apple cider vinegar, red wine vinegar, balsamic vinegar or white wine vinegar.

Salad toppings – use chopped walnuts, sliced almonds or seeds.

Sandwiches

Use wholegrain, seeded or sprouted breads and wraps. Add your choice of veggies and protein.

Some great fillings to try are:

- cold poached salmon and spinach,

- chicken, avocado and basil,

- goats cheese with roast veggies and avocado,

- spinach, grated carrots, cucumber and hummus

Snack Attacks

Snack on healthy food. It's really important to prepare snack foods in advance so when you get a hunger pang, you can quickly reach for a healthy snack. Pre – peel and cut fruits and veggies and keep them in the fridge for when you are hungry.

Savoury Snack Ideas:

Feta cheese cubes and olives

Marinated feta and olives - you can marinate your own cubes of feta cheese and green or/and black olives in extra virgin olive oil. Add your choice of raw garlic cloves or lemon slices. Choose herbs like basil, rosemary or thyme to infuse the oil and add flavour. Store them in glass jars in the fridge.

Warm olives – olives warmed through in olive oil that has been infused with spices and herbs.

- Olives

- Spices: chilli, fennel seeds, coriander seeds

- Herbs: rosemary sprigs, thyme,

- Others: sliced garlic, lemon or orange zest

Use 1 tbsp. of olive oil for one cup of olives of your choice. Heat the olive oil in a small pan on low heat for a minute, then add your choice of herbs/spices and let their flavor infuse the oil for another minute. Add the olives and heat through gently for a few minutes.

Whole grain or seeded crisp breads, flatbreads or crackers – eat with dips, cheese or olives

Kale Chips - a delicious alternative to fatty crisps and easy to make. Use a bag of curly kale and start by roughly tearing the leaves off their stems. Coat the kale leaves in 2 tbsp of olive oil by tossing both ingredients in a bowl. Add some salt. Spread the leaves out onto a couple of baking trays. Bake at 300 C for 10- 15 minutes until the leaves are crisp.

Roasted pumpkin seeds –Preheat oven to 150 C. Put 100 g of pumpkin seeds in a bowl and mix in 1 tsp of olive oil and a pinch of salt. Line a baking tray with tin foil and spread the seeds out onto the tray. Bake for 15- 20 min until the seeds start to brown. Keep checking them and stir them about as they have a tendency to burn easily.

Air popped popcorn - you can pop popcorn kernels on the stove top in a large pot without using oil as long as you keep shaking kernels around frequently until they have popped or use a popcorn machine(air popper). Flavour with a small amount of sea salt or parmesan shavings, herbs, or cayenne pepper.

Boiled eggs – sprinkle with cayenne pepper

Raw vegetables crudites – In advance prepare veggies to snack on. Tasty choices - (carrots, peppers, broccoli, cauliflower, celery, sugarsnap peas, celery, cucumber are a few good choices). Preferably make your own dips using beans, pulses and veggies i.e. guacamole, hummus, white bean dips.

Sweet Snack Ideas

Nut butters (almond/cashew) on apple or banana slices

High quality dark chocolate buttons

Unsweetened dried fruit with nuts/seeds

Popcorn - Try adding shavings of dark chocolate, or cinnamon to air-popped popcorn

Apple or pear slices with thin slices of parmesan cheese

Drinks

Teas –Swap to herbal teas.

Green teas – if you find green tea too strong a taste to enjoy, try green tea bags which are combined with lemon as it cuts the strong taste of green tea which some people find hard to consume. Green tea also comes combined with peppermint, cranberry and other flavours.

Other herbal teas include peppermint, chamomile, ginger, nettle and dandelion. There are loads of choices out there.

Make your own fresh herbal teas – steep fresh mint leaves in hot water. I love the combination of fresh lemon balm leaves and mint leaves. Try fresh grated ginger with lemon and sweeten with a bit of honey if needed.

Milk

Try swapping cow's milk for goat's milk. If you want to reduce your dairy intake try almond or rice milk.

Alcohol

Alcohol should really be avoided but if you do drink alcohol the best choice is red wine (preferably organic) but limited to 1-2 glasses per day. Red wine has beneficial antioxidant activity.

Flavourings

Adding flavour is really important if you want to make your meals tasty.

Salt - Use sea salt or Himalayan salt as it is rich in minerals and less refined than classic table salt

Sugar: Use natural sources to sweeten your food. You can use mashed figs and dates, orange juice, unsweetened fruit compotes or small amounts of maple syrup, agave nectar, or raw unpasteurized/organic honey.

Spice it up: Be generous when using herb and spices to flavour your foods

Spices: black pepper, cinnamon, curry powder, cayenne pepper, chilli, ginger, turmeric,

Herbs: basil, cardamom, chives, oregano, parsley, rosemary, sage, thyme

Find recipes where you can make your own home-made dressings for salads, marinades for your meat and dips for your veggies.

In a Nutshell

To be in control of your symptoms, you need to follow a diet which rich in anti–inflammatory foods. Eat more fruit and vegetables, fish, wholegrains, nuts and seeds as they are rich in anti-oxidants and essential nutrients. Eat foods that lower your glycemic load to balance your blood sugar levels. Eliminate toxic and allergic foods from your diet and support your body with healing herbal supplements.

Step 1. Reduce foods that promote inflammation in the body

- Avoid Refined carbs such as white flour, white rice and pasta

- Avoid Coffee, Black tea, Soft Drinks and Alcohol

- Avoid Processed Foods, Additives/ Preservatives and Sweeteners

- Avoid Trans-fats

- Reduce your meat intake

Step 2. Introduce foods that are anti-inflammatory into your diet

- Eat a variety of vegetables and fruits

- Eat Omega- 3 rich foods

- Eat good Oils/Fats - stick to the healthy ones: omega 3's, extra-virgin olive oil, coconut, walnut, avocado and grapeseed oils

- Eat smaller quantities of meat and choose organic or free range meats

- Eat wholegrains

- Prepare meals and snacks that incorporate the anti-arthritic superfoods

- Reduce the cooking temperature of fish and meats to reduce AGES

Step 3. Keep your blood sugar levels balanced

- Choose foods that are low-medium on the glycemic index

- Slow down insulin spikes by adding fat or protein to carbs to reduce sudden rises in blood sugar levels.

- Reduce your sugar intake: stick to natural sweeteners but in limited quantities

Step 4. Eliminate anti-arthritic foods

Sometimes simply eating better can be enough to make a significant change to your symptoms and that's great. However you could be intolerant to certain foods that worsen your symptoms.

- Keep a food diary and look for a link between certain foods and a flare-up in your symptoms

- Eliminate unhealthy fats, processed foods and refined carbohydrates

- Use the elimination diet to test suspected food groups

Step 5 - Add herbs and supplements that reduce joint inflammation and support cartilage

Adding herbal supplements is often an effective way in supporting your body's healing mechanisms. Long-term use of NSAID's and analgesics are associated with unpleasant and sometimes serious side effects. Research has found supplements that can be beneficial in easing symptoms, repairing cartilage and preventing further joint and cartilage damage.

- Research the benefits of the supplements you want to try.

- Find sound scientific evidence which demonstrate the effectiveness herbal supplements. Randomized, double-blinded trials and evidence based reviews are

- Check with you GP before you start a supplement if you are on any other medications as herbal supplements can interact and affect the way your medication works.

- Try one supplement at a time

- Record your symptoms, giving each supplement 2-3 months to take effect

I hope that you have found the information in this ebook useful and that it has motivated you to change your eating and lifestyle habits to help you ease your symptoms. You can have control over your health and you can affect your body's healing mechanisms so that they work at their most efficient and optimal levels to keep you healthy and feeling better.

Remember .... Eat well to Stay Well

References

1. http://articles.mercola.com/sites/articles/archive/2011/01/31/curcumin-relieves-pain-and-inflammation-for-osteoarthritis-patients.aspx

2. Sheild, MJ "Anti-inflammatory drugs and their effects on Cartilage synthesis and renal function" Eur J Rheumatol Inflam 13 (1993): 7-16

3. Hauser, R.A The Acceleration of Articular Cartilage Degeneration in Osteoarthritis by Nonsteroidal Anti-inflammatory Drugs *Journal of Prolotherapy*.2010;(2)1:305-322

4. http://arthritis.about.com/cs/steroids/a/corticosteroids_2.htm

5. http://www.arthritisresearchuk.org/arthritis-information/drugs/painkillers/paracetamol.aspx

6. Benefits and Risks of Opioids in Arthritis Management by Michael Clark, M.D., M.P.H. http://www.hopkinsarthritis.org/patient-corner/disease-management/benefits-and-risks-of-opioids-for-chronic-pain-management/

7. http://www.arthritisresearchuk.org/arthritis-information/drugs/painkillers/opioid-analgesics/types-of-opiod-analgesics.aspx

8. Jang, H and Serra, C (2014), Nutrition, Epigenetics and Diseases, Clin Nutr Res. Jan 2014; 3(1): 1–8.

9. Hunter, P, The inflammation theory of disease: The growing realization that chronic inflammation is crucial in many diseases opens new avenues for treatment **DOI** 10.1038/embor.2012.142

10. Yudoh, K et al, Potential Involvement of Oxidative Stress in Cartilage Senescence and Development of Osteoarthritis: Oxidative Stress Induces Chondrocyte Telomere Instability and Downregulation of Chondrocyte Function; Arthritis Research & Therapy, Jan 2005

11. Holt, SHA, Brand-Miller, JC. International tables of glycemic index and glycemic load values. Am J Clin Nutr 2002;62: 5–56.

12. Adam O, Beringer C, Kless T, Lemmen C, Adam A, Wiseman M, Adam P, Klimmek R, Forth W. Anti-inflammatory effects of a low arachidonic acid diet and fish oil in patients with rheumatoid arthritis. Rheumatol Int. 2003 Jan;23(1):27-36. Epub 2002 Sep 6.

13. Tucker KL, Morita K, Qiao N, Hannan MT, Cupples LA, and Kiel DP. Colas, but not other carbonated beverages, are associated with low bone mineral density in older women: The Framingham Osteoporosis Study. Am J Clin Nutr. 2006 Oct; 84(4):936-42.

14. Neblett, A, Arthritis and Alcohol: A Bad Mix http://www.qualityhealth.com/arthritis-articles/arthritis-alcohol-bad-mix

15. Childers N.F. and Margoles M.S., An apparent relation of nightshades to arthritis, Journal of Neurological and Orthopaedic Medical Surgery, 1993: 12-227-331

16. Childers N.F. A relationship of arthritis to the Solanaceae (nightshades). J Intern Acad Prev Med 1979; 7:31-37

17. http://www.medicalnewstoday.com/releases/9463.php

18. Mori TA et al 2004, Omega-3 fatty acids and inflammation. Curr Atheroscler Rep. 2004 Nov;6(6):461-7.

19. Surette, M.E, The science behind dietary omega-3 fatty acids CMAJ, 2008 vol. 178 no. 2

20. http://www.chiro.org/nutrition/FULL/Chronic_Joint_Pain.shtml

21. Miggiano GA et al 2005 Diet, nutrition and rheumatoid arthritis. Clin Ter. 2005 May-Jun;156 (3):115-23.

22. http://www.whfoods.com/genpage.php?tname=george&dbid=75

23. http://www.nlm.nih.gov/medlineplus/druginfo/natural/993.html fish

24. http://umm.edu/health/medical/altmed/supplement/omega3-fatty-acids

25. http://www.arthritisresearchuk.org/arthritis-information/complementary-and-alternative-medicines/cam-report/complementary-medicines-for-rheumatoid-arthritis/vitamins-ace/trials-for-oa.aspx

26. http://www.umm.edu/altmed/articles/vitamin-c-000339.htm#ixzz1vD2aNTSo

27. Arthritis Today: The Right Amount of Vitamin C, http://www.arthritistoday.org/what-you-can-do/eating-well/vitamins-and-minerals/vitamin-c-amount.php

28. Xu H, Watkins BA, Seifert MF. Vitamin E stimulates trabecular bone formation and alters epiphyseal cartilage morphometry. Calcif Tissu Int 1995;57:293–300

29. www.selenium.co.za

30. King, D.E. MD, Effect of a High-Fiber Diet vs a Fiber-Supplemented Diet on C-Reactive Protein Level Archives of Internal Medicine, March 2007; 12;167(5):502-6

31. American Institute for Cancer Research (AICR) International Conference on Food, Nutrition and Cancer, Nov. 2004

32. Boots AW, Haenen GR, Bast A. Health effects of quercetin: from antioxidant to nutraceutical. *Eur J Pharmacol*. 2008;582(2-3):325-37.

33. Davidson RK, Jupp O, De Ferrars R, Kay CD, Culley KL, Norton R, Driscoll C, Vincent TL, Donell ST, Bao Y and Clark IM; "Sulforaphane represses matrix-degrading proteases and protects cartilage from destruction in vitro and in vivo"; Arthritis & Rheumatism published online 27 August 2013; DOI: 10.1002/art.38133

34. Journal of Natural Products, January 29, 1999.

35. Howatson, G., McHugh, M.P., Hill, J., Brouner, J., Jewell, A., van Someren, K.A., Shave, R. Howatson, S.A. (2010). The effects of a tart cherry juice supplement on muscle damage, inflammation, oxidative stress and recovery following Marathon running. Scandinavian Journal of Medicine and Science in Sports, 20, 843-52

36. Cush JJ. Baylor Research Institute, pilot study on tart cherry and osteoarthritis of the knees, 2007

37. Kuehl KS, Elliot DL, Sleigh A, Smith J. Efficacy of tart cherry juice to reduce inflammation biomarkers among women with inflammatory osteoarthritis. J Food Stud. 2012;1:14-25

38. Di Giuseppe R, Di Castelnuovo A et al, "Regular consumption of dark chocolate is associated with low serum concentrations of C-reactive protein in a healthy Italian population" J Nutr. 2008 Oct;138(10):1939-45.

39. Williams, F.M.K et al, " Dietary garlic and hip osteoarthritis: evidence of a protective effect and putative mechanism of action." BMC Musculoskeletal Disorders 2010, 11:280

40. Altman RD, Marcussen KC. Effects of a ginger extract on knee pain in patients with osteoarthritis, Arthritis Rheum. 2001 Nov;44(11):2531-8.

41. Ahmed, S, et al. Green Tea Polyphenol Epigallocatechin-3-gallate (EGCG) Differentially Inhibits Interleukin-1-Induced Expression of Matrix Metalloproteinase-1 and -13 in Human Chondrocytes. J Pharmacol Exp Ther 2004;308(2):767-773

42. Adcocks, C, et al. Catechins from gree tea (*Camellia sinensis*) inhibit bovine and human cartilage protoglycan and type II collagen degradation in vitro. 2002 J Nutr;132(3):341-6

43. http://www.umm.edu/altmed/articles/green-tea-000255.htm#ixzz1vD7MzXZo

44. Isaacs CE, Litov RE, Marie P, Thormar H. Addition of lipases to infant formulas produces antiviral and antibacterial activity, Journal of Nutritional Biochemistry, 1992;3:304-308

45. Matsumoto, M., Takeru Kobayashi, T., Akio Takenakaand, A. and Hisao Itabashi, H. Defaunation Effects of Medium Chain Fatty Acids and Their Derivatives on Goat Rumen Protozoa, The Journal of General Applied Microbiology, Vol. 37, No. 5 (1991) pp.439-445.

46. St-Onge MP and Jones PJ. Greater rise in fat oxidation with medium-chain triglyceride consumption relative to long-chain triglyceride is associated with lower initial body weight and greater loss of subcutaneous adipose tissue, International Journal of Obesity & Related Metabolic Disorders, 2003 Dec;27(12):1565-71

47. Beauchamp GK et al. Phytochemistry : ibuprofen-like activity in extra-virgin olive oil. Nature 2005; 437:45-6

48. http://www.arthritistoday.org/what-you-can-do/eating-well/healthy-foods/healthy-oils.php

49. http://www.ncbi.nlm.nih.gov/pubmed/12975635

50. Andrew Weil, MD. Can Herbs Combat Inflammation? http://www.drweil.com/drw/u/QAA142972/Anti-Inflammatory-Herbs.com

51. Edirisinghe I,Banaszewski J, Capozzo J et al, "Strawberry anthocyanin and its association with postprandial inflammation and insulin "Br J Nutr. 2011 Sep; 106(6):913-22

52. Aggarwal BB, Sung B. Pharmacological basis for the role of curcumin in chronic diseases: an age-old spice with modern targets. Trends Pharmacol Sci..2009;30:85-94.

53. Akhtar NM, Naseer R, Farooqi AZ, Aziz W, Nazir M, Oral enzyme combination versus diclofenac in the treatment of osteoarthritis of the knee--a double-blind prospective randomized study. Clin Rheumatol. 2004 Oct;23(5):410-5.

54. Belcaro G, Cesarone MR, Dugall M, Pellegrini L, Ledda A, Grossi MG, Togni S, Appendino G. Product-evaluation registry of Meriva®, curcumin-phosphatidylcholine complex, for the complementary management of osteoarthritis. *PanMinerva Med.* 2010;52 (Suppl. 1 to No. 1):55-62

55. Shoba G, Joy D, Joseph T, Majeed M, Rajendran R, Srinivas PS. Influence of piperine on the pharmacokinetics of curcumin in animals and human volunteers. Planta Med. 1998 May;64(4):353-6

56. McCarty MF, Russell AL. Niacinamide therapy for osteoarthritis--does it inhibit nitric oxide synthase

57. http://www.arthritisresearchuk.org/arthritis-information/complementary-and-alternative-medicines/cam-report/complementary-medicines-for-rheumatoid-arthritis/vitamins-b-complex/trials-for-oa.aspx

58. http://umm.edu/health/medical/altmed/supplement/vitamin-b3-niacin

59. http://www.whfoods.com/genpage.php?tname=nutrient&dbid=83

60. Haroon M, Bond U, Quillinan N, Phelan MJ and Regan MJ. The prevalence of vitamin D deficiency in consecutive new patients seen over a 6-month period in general rheumatology clinics. Clin Rheumatol. 2011 Jun;30(6):789-94

61. Mouyis, M, Ostor, AJ, Crisp, AJ, et al. Hypovitaminosis D among rheumatology outpatients in clinical practice. Rheumatology (Oxford) 2008;47(9):1348-51

62. http://ods.od.nih.gov/factsheets/VitaminD-HealthProfessional/

63. Barclay, A.W., Petocz P., McMillan-Price, J., Flood, V.M., Prvan T., Paul Mitchell, P., and Brand-Miller, J.C. Glycemic index, glycemic load, and chronic disease risk. American Journal of Clinical Nutrition March 2008, Vol. 87, No. 3, [627-637]

64. The Glycemic Index, www.dlife.com

66. Kate Hicks, Gillian Hart, "Role for food-specific IgG-based elimination diets", Nutrition & Food Science, 2008, Vol. 38 Iss: 5, pp.404 – 416

67. http://www.universitynutrition.co.uk/articles/elimination-diets/

68. www.uccs.edu/.../peakfood/hlthTopics/Allergy%20Elimination%20Diet.pdf

69.http://www.natrx.com.au/epages/nms.sf/en_AU/?ObjectPath=/Shops/nms/Products/9008/SubProducts/9008-0001

70. Gundermann KJ, Müller J. Phytodolor--effects and efficacy of a herbal medicine. Wien Med Wochenschr. 2007;157(13-14):343-7.

71. Complementary and alternative medicines for the treatment of rheumatoid arthritis, osteoarthritis and fibromyalgia: A report by the Arthritis Research Campaign. Published online February 10 2009 http://www.arthritisresearchuk.org/

72. www.pachealth.co.nz/_res/docs/Flordis/Phytodolor.pdf· PDF file

73. http://arthritis.about.com/od/same/a/whatissame.htm

74. Najm, W.I. et al. S-Adenosyl methionine (SAM-e) versus celecoxib for the treatment of osteoarthritis symptoms: A double-blind cross-over trial. BMC Musculoskeletal Disorders, Feb 2004. http://www.biomedcentral.com/1471-2474/5/6

75. http://www.lef.org/protocols/immune_connective_joint/osteoarthritis_01.htm

76. Safety and efficacy of S-adenosylmethionine (SAM-e) for osteoarthritis. Soeken KL et al. The Journal of Family Practice. May 2002.

77. http://www.nhs.uk/news/2008/05May/Pages/Rosehipforosteoarthritispain.aspx

78. Cohen M. Rosehip - an evidence based herbal medicine for inflammation and arthritis. aust fam physician 2012 Jul;41(7):495-8

79. Warholm O, Skaar S, Hedman E, Mølmen HM, Eik L. The effects of a standardized herbal remedy made from a subtype of Rosa canina in patients with osteoarthritis: a double-blind, randomized, placebo-controlled clinical trial. Curr Ther Res Clin Exp 2003;64:21–31

80. Winther, K. Apel, K and Thomsborg,G. 'A powder made from seeds and shells of a rose-hip subspecies (Rosa canina l.) reduces symptoms of knee and hip osteoarthritis: A randomized, double-blind, placebo-controlled clinical trial.' Scandinavian Journal Rheumatology, 34:302-308, July - August 2005

81. Christensen R, Bartels EM, Altman RD et al. Does the hip powder of Rosa canina (rosehip) reduce pain in osteoarthritis patients? - a meta-analysis of randomized controlled trials. Osteoarthritis Cartilage 2008; 16: 965-972.

82. http://www.rxlist.com/rose_hip-page3/supplements.htm

83. http://www.webmd.com/vitamins-and-supplements/rosehip-uses-and-risks

84. http://altmedicine.about.com/od/arthritis/a/avocado_soybean_arthritis.htm

85. Maheu E, Mazieres B, Valat JP, Loyau G, Le L, X, Bourgeois P, et al. Symptomatic efficacy of avocado/soybean unsaponifiables in the treatment of osteoarthritis of the knee and hip: a prospective, randomized, double-blind, placebo-controlled, multicenter clinical trial with a six-month treatment period and a two-month followup demonstrating a persistent effect. Arthritis Rheum 1998 Jan;41(1):81-91

86. Ameye L.G. and Chee W.S.S, Osteoarthritis and nutrition. From nutraceuticals to functional foods: a systematic review of the scientific evidence, Arthritis Research & Therapy 2006, 8:R127

87. Appelboom T, Schuermans J, Verbruggen G, Henrotin Y, Reginster JY. Symptoms modifying effect of avocado/soybean unsaponifiables (ASU) in knee osteoarthritis. A double blind, prospective, placebo-controlled study. Scand J Rheumatol 2001;30(4):242-7

88. http://howdrugs.com/avocado/

89. http://www.webmd.com/vitamins-supplements/ingredientmono-890-AVOCADO.aspx?activeIngredi

90. Cisar, P. et al, " Effect of Pine Bark Extract (Pycnogenol) on Symptoms of Knee Osteoarthritis"; Phytotherapy Research, Aug 2008

91. Belcaro G, Cesarone MR, Errichi S, Zulli C, ErrichiBM, Vinciguerra G et al. Treatment of osteoarthritis with Pycnogenol. The SVOS (San Valentino Osteo-arthrosis Study). Evaluation of signs, symptoms, physical performance and vascular aspects. Phytotherapy Research 2008; 22(4):518–23

92. http://www.nlm.nih.gov/medlineplus/druginfo/natural/1019.html

93. Black C, Clar C, Henderson R, MacEachern C, McNamee P, Quayyum Z, Royle P, Thomas S The clinical effectiveness of glucosamine and chondroitin supplements in slowing or arresting progression, Health Technology Assessment 2009; 13(52): 1-148

94. Qui GX, et al. Efficacy and Safety of Glucosamine Sulfate Versus Ibuprofen in Patients with Knee Osteoarthritis. Arzneimittelforschung. May1998;48(5):469-74

95. Gruenwald J, Petzold E, Busch R, Petzold HP, Graubaum HJ. Effect of glucosamine sulfate with or without omega-3 fatty acids in patients with osteoarthritis. Adv Ther. 2009 26:858-71. Epub 2009 Sep 4

96. http://www.arthritistoday.org/arthritis-treatment/natural-and-alternative-treatments/supplements-and-herbs/supplement-guide/glucosamine.php

97. Bucsi L, Poor G. Efficacy and tolerability of oral chondroitin sulfate as a symptomatic slow-acting drug for osteoarthritis (SYSADOA) in the treatment of knee osteoarthritis. *Osteoarthritis Cartilage.* 1998;6(suppl A):31-36.

98. Verbruggen G, Goemaere S, Veys EM. Chondroitin sulfate: S/DMOAD (structure/disease modifying anti-osteoarthritis drug) in the treatment of finger joint OA. *Osteoarthritis Cartilage.* 1998;6(suppl A):37-38

99. http://nccam.nih.gov/research/results/gait/qa.htm

100. http://www.nlm.nih.gov/medlineplus/druginfo/natural/744.html

101. Kim LS, Axelrod LJ, Howard P, Buratovich N, Waters RF. Efficacy of methylsulfonylmethane (MSM) in osteoarthritis pain of the knee: a pilot clinical trial, Osteoarthritis Cartilage, 2006 Mar;14(3):286-94

102. http://www.webmd.com/vitamins-supplements/ingredientmono-522-MSM%20(METHYLSULFONYLMETHANE).aspx?activeIngredientId=522&activeIngredientName=MSM%20(METHYLSULFONYLMETHANE)

103. Poulsen et al, Advanced glycation end products in food and their effects on health. Food and chemical toxicology vol 60 oct 2013 10-37

104. Uribarri, J. et al., Advanced glycation end products in foods and a practical guide to their reduction in the diet. *Journal of the American Dietetic Association* 2010 Jun;110(6):911-916.e12.

Printed in Great Britain
by Amazon